Advances in Intelligent Systems and Computing

Volume 1028

The series "Advances in Intelligent Systems and Computing" contains publications on theory, applications, and design methods of Intelligent Systems and Intelligent Computing. Virtually all disciplines such as engineering, natural sciences, computer and information science, ICT, economics, business, e-commerce, environment, healthcare, life science are covered. The list of topics spans all the areas of modern intelligent systems and computing such as: computational intelligence, soft computing including neural networks, fuzzy systems, evolutionary computing and the fusion of these paradigms, social intelligence, ambient intelligence, computational neuroscience, artificial life, virtual worlds and society, cognitive science and systems, Perception and Vision, DNA and immune based systems, self-organizing and adaptive systems, e-Learning and teaching, human-centered and human-centric computing, recommender systems, intelligent control, robotics and mechatronics including human-machine teaming, knowledge-based paradigms, learning paradigms, machine ethics, intelligent data analysis, knowledge management, intelligent agents, intelligent decision making and support, intelligent network security, trust management, interactive entertainment, Web intelligence and multimedia.

The publications within "Advances in Intelligent Systems and Computing" are primarily proceedings of important conferences, symposia and congresses. They cover significant recent developments in the field, both of a foundational and applicable character. An important characteristic feature of the series is the short publication time and world-wide distribution. This permits a rapid and broad dissemination of research results.

** Indexing: The books of this series are submitted to ISI Proceedings, EI-Compendex, DBLP, SCOPUS, Google Scholar and Springerlink **

More information about this series at http://www.springer.com/series/11156

Martin Lames · Alexander Danilov ·
Egor Timme · Yuri Vassilevski
Editors

Proceedings of the 12th International Symposium on Computer Science in Sport (IACSS 2019)

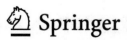 Springer

Editors
Martin Lames
Faculty of Sports and Health Sciences
Technical University Munich
Munich, Bayern, Germany

Alexander Danilov
Marchuk Institute of Numerical Mathematics
Russian Academy of Science
Moscow, Russia

Egor Timme
Moscow Centre for Advanced Sports
Technology
Moscow, Russia

Yuri Vassilevski
Marchuk Institute of Numerical Mathematics
Russian Academy of Science
Moscow, Russia

ISSN 2194-5357 ISSN 2194-5365 (electronic)
Advances in Intelligent Systems and Computing
ISBN 978-3-030-35047-5 ISBN 978-3-030-35048-2 (eBook)
https://doi.org/10.1007/978-3-030-35048-2

This Springer imprint is published by the registered company Springer Nature Switzerland AG
The registered company address is: Gewerbestrasse 11, 6330 Cham, Switzerland

Preface

The 12th International Symposium of Computer Science in Sports (IACSS 2019) took place July 8–10, 2019, at Marchuk Institute of Numerical Mathematics of the Russian Academy of Science and the Moscow Center of Advanced Sports Technologies (MCAST), both situated in Moscow, Russia. The symposium continued a tradition of conferences starting in 1997 at Cologne, Germany, which were held biennially and traveled through many countries and continents since then.

Though the topics of the presentations have changed, the aims of the symposium are still the same. The symposium engages in building links between computer science and sports science and showcases a wide variety of applications of computer science techniques to a wide number of problems in sports and exercise sciences. Moreover, it provides a platform for researchers in both computer science and sports science for mutual understanding, discussing the respective ideas, and promoting cross-disciplinary research.

This year the symposium addressed the following topics:

Computer Science:

- Modeling and Simulation
- Sports Data Acquisition Systems
- Image and Video Processing
- Sports Data Analysis
- Machine Learning and Data Mining
- Visualization and Visual Analytics
- Presentation, Communication
- Decision Support
- Robotics
- Virtual Reality
- Digital Games

Sports and Exercise Science:

- Biomechanics and Neuromuscular Control
- Exercise Physiology and Sports Medicine

- Performance Development and Analysis
- Training, Coaching, and Feedback
- Modeling of Adaptation, Fatigue, and Performance
- Optimization of Strategies for Best Performance
- Movement, Motor Control, and Learning
- Sports Management

We received 41 papers submissions and all of them underwent strict and blind reviews by the Program Committee. At least two reviewers commented on each paper, resulting in an acceptance rate of 59%. Authors of the 24 accepted papers were asked to revise their papers carefully according to the detailed comments so that they all meet the expected high quality of an international conference.

Six keynote speakers and the authors of the accepted papers presented their contributions in the above topics during the 3-day event.

A get-together reception, a guided tour through MCAST, and a boat trip on the Moskva River with the conference dinner were the highlights of the social program.

We thank Springer Publishers for providing the opportunity of continuing the tradition that started with Loughborough 2015 and was continued with Konstanz 2017, of publishing the conference proceedings in their series "Advances in Intelligent Systems and Computing."

We thank the participants for coming to Moscow and hope that it was an enjoyable and fruitful event for all participants. We also thank the Program Committee members, the Local Organization Committee members, the reviewers, the invited speakers, and the presenters for their contributions to make the event a success.

Martin Lames
Alexander Danilov
Egor Timme
Yuri Vassilevski

Organization

Program Chairs

Martin Lames	TU München, Germany
Alexander Danilov	Marchuk Institute, Russian Academy of Sciences, Moscow
Egor Timme	Moscow Center of Advanced Sports Technologies
Yuri Vassilevski	Marchuk Institute, Russian Academy of Sciences, Moscow

Program Committee

Egor Akimov	Akivino, Sports High Performance Corp., USA
Arnold Baca	University of Vienna, Austria
Olga Bazanova	Institute of Physiology and Basic Medicine, Russia
Alexey Bogomolov	Federal Medical Biological Agency, Russia
Thierry Busso	Université Jean Monnet, Saint-Etienne, France
Dmitry Dagaev	Higher School of Economics, Russia
Jürgen Edelmann-Nusser	Otto-von-Guericke University Magdeburg, Germany
Hayri Ertan	Eskişehir Technical University, Turkey
Ewan Griffith	Swansea University, UK
Alena Grushko	Lomonosov Moscow State University, Russia
Otto Kolbinger	Technical University of Munich, Germany
Nikolay Kulemin	Federal Medical Biological Agency, Russia
Rajesh Kumar	Osmania University, Hyderabad, India
Vladimir Kurashvili	The Federal Training Center of Sports Reserve, Russia

Martin Lames	Technical University of Munich, Germany
Daniel Link	Technical University of Munich, Germany
Keith Lyons	University of Canberra, Australia
Chikara Miyaji	Japanese Institute of Sport, Japan
Jürgen Perl	University of Mainz, Germany
Oleg Popov	Russian State University SCOLIPE, Russia
Tiago Russomanno	University of Brasilia, Brazil
Dietmar Saupe	Universität Konstanz, Germany
Michael Stöckl	University of Vienna, Austria
Egor Timme	Russian Association of Computer Science in Sport, Russia
Josef Wiemeyer	Technical University of Darmstadt, Germany
Kerstin Witte	Otto-von-Guericke University Magdeburg, Germany
Hui Zhang	Zhejiang University, Hangzhou, China

Invited Keynote Speakers

Cathy Craig	CEO/Founder INCISIV Ltd., Belfast, Northern Ireland
Jesse Davis	Department of Computer Science, KU Leuven, Belgium
Stuart Morgan	La Trobe University, AIS, Canberra, Australia
Sergey Simakov	Sechenov University, Moscow, Russia
Mikhail A. Vinogradov	MCAST, ROC, Moscow, Russia
Yingcai Wu	Zhejiang University, Hangzhou, China

IACSS Organizing Committee

Martin Lames (President of the Symposium)	Technical University of Munich, Germany
Philipp Kornfeind	University of Vienna, Austria
Michael Stöckl	University of Vienna, Austria
Hui Zhang	Zhejiang University, Hangzhou, China

Local Organizing Committee

Yuri Vassilevski (Co-chair of the Local Organizing Committee)	Marchuk Institute of Numerical Mathematics, Russia
Kadriya Akhmerova (Co-chair of the Local Organizing Committee)	Moscow Center of Advanced Sport Technologies, Russia
Alexander Danilov (Secretary of the Symposium)	Marchuk Institute of Numerical Mathematics, Russia

Egor Timme   Russian Association of Computer Science
                                         in Sport, Russia
Philipp Kopylov   Sechenov University, Russia
Marina Izvekova   Sport Science Association, Russia

Invited Lectures

Using Virtual Reality to Understand and Improve Decision-Making in Sport: What We Need to Consider

Cathy Craig[1,2]

[1]Ulster University, Coleraine, N. Ireland
[2]INCISIV Ltd., 18 Ormeau Avenue, Belfast, N. Ireland
cathy@incisiv.tech

Abstract. In sport, it has often been said that the technical, tactical, and physical differences between players are often minimal, but the key thing that separates the best from the rest is a player's ability to make winning decisions under pressure. In the age of the quantified athlete, there are many technologies out there that tell us something about the physical (e.g., GPS) or physiological (e.g., heart rate) aspects of performance, but there are no technologies that can tell us about a player's psychology and their ability to make the right decision, at the right time and execute it in the right way.

When adopting a technology to study decision-making, it is important that it can reproduce the immersive and interactive experience a player would have on the sporting field. Virtual reality technology offers an exciting new way of studying decision-making in sport where the user can behave in the virtual world as they do in the real world (Craig 2014). The versatility of this technology means it can be easily applied to many different sports (e.g., rugby (Brault et al. 2012), soccer (Dessing and Craig 2010), cricket (Dhawan et al. 2016)). As a versatile method-ological tool, it gives the user complete control over complex environmental conditions and allows for an in-depth analysis of the user's responses. The advent of new hardware solutions such as the HTC Vive and Oculus Rift is now making immersive, interactive virtual reality much more mainstream and is opening up exciting new opportunities to use this technology in sports in a very practical way. The low-cost technology with very reliable motion tracking means it can be used to profile player performance, provide opportunities for teams to train smarter and protect players from injury. This new technology can help add value to the coaching process and offer new insight into player performance.

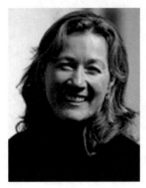

Bio. Cathy Craig is the recognized go-to global expert in using virtual reality to understand decision-making in sport. The caliber of her research is evidenced by over 80 research publications (>2860 citations, H-index = 32; i10 = 54; source Google Scholar) published in top quality journals (e.g., Nature, IEEE) that include 90 different co-authors from nine different countries in a range of multi-disciplinary areas (e.g., computer science, engineering). After 20 years in academia, she has founded INCISIV Ltd. to translate her know-how into practical applications.

Assessing the Performances of Soccer Players

Jesse Davis

Department of Computer Science, KU Leuven, Belgium
jesse.davis@cs.kuleuven.be

Abstract. A key question within sports analytics is how to analyze match data in order to objectively assess a player's performance during a match. In this talk, I will describe our recent research on trying to address this question for soccer. Our approach involves two components. First, our mental pressure model assigns a pressure level to each game situation by considering both the match context as well as the current game state. Second, we use machine-learned models to evaluate three aspects of each on-the-ball action performed by a player: the choice of action, the execution of the chosen action, and the action's expected contribution to the scoreline. This enables comparing the player's performances across different levels of mental pressure. I will show our approach's ability to provide actionable insights for several different use cases.

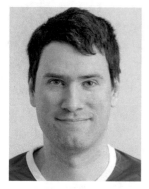

Bio. Jesse Davis is an associate professor in the Department of Computer Science at KU Leuven in Belgium. He received his bachelor's degree from Williams College (USA) and his masters' and Ph.D. from the University of Wisconsin–Madison (USA). He completed a three-year postdoc at the University of Washington (USA). He is also a co-founder of Activ84Health, an awarding-winning start-up whose mission is to motivate elderly individuals to remain physically active.

Harvesting Sports Science Insight with Computer Vision

Stuart Morgan

Australian Institute of Sport, Canberra, Australia
Stuart.Morgan@ausport.gov.au

Abstract. A battleground exists between countries on a technological front, where novel and innovative technologies are seen to provide elite athletes with a small edge that could be the difference for an athlete to win (or not win) a gold medal. In this presentation, we will discuss how and why is computer vision useful in the "real" world of Olympic sport, and how these technologies are being employed to enable athletes to perform consistently at the highest level. This presentation will explore ways that computer vision technology is deployed in high-performance sport, and how the decisions made by coaches can be augmented by machine learning and computer vision.

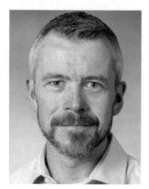

Bio. Stuart Morgan is the Head of Computer Vision and Machine Learning at the Australian Institute of Sport, Associate Professor in Computer Science at La Trobe University, and Adjunct Associate Professor in Computer Science at Queensland University of Technology. He has 18 years of experience in computer sciences and sports analytics in high-performance sport, including work with numerous high profile international teams at World Championships and Olympic Games.

Mathematical Modeling of the Cardiovascular and Respiratory Systems in Sport

Sergey Simakov[1,2]

[1]Moscow Institute of Physics and Technology,
 9 Institutskii Lane, Dolgoprudny, Russia, 141701
[2]Sechenov University, 19/1 Bol'shaya Pirogovskaya,
 Moscow, Russia, 119146
 simakov.ss@mipt.ru

Abstract. The reduced order mathematical models of the cardiovascular and respiratory systems will be presented. They include various physiological features such as regulatory and autoregulatory responses, effect of muscle contraction, and venous valves function. The 1D network models of the cardiovascular and respiratory systems describe the blood flow and respiratory gas flow in the large and medium vessels and bronchial tubes. The lumped parameter model is used for the description of the transport of respiratory gases in the organism and metabolic processes over a long time (up to several hours). Some applications to the sports science will be presented including blood flow variations depending on the stride frequency and assessment of the effectiveness of the athlete depending on his performance in the laboratory conditions.

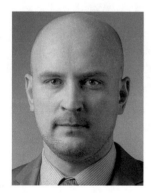

Bio. Sergey Simakov is an associate professor in the Department of Computational Physics of (MIPT) in Russia. He received his bachelor's, masters', and Ph.D. degree from MIPT (Russia). He was rewarded by Award Best Young Teacher from V. Potanin Foundation in 2009, by Award of the President of the Russian Federation for Young Scientists in 2012. He is a partner of NESA, an expert of RACS. He was the guest editor of the Journal of Mathematical Modeling for Natural Phenomena and Computer Research and Modeling and editor of the volume "Smart Modeling for Engineering Systems", Springer-Verlag, Germany. He supervised two Ph.D. students. His main research interests are computational mathematics, numerical methods, modeling of the wave processes in a network, modeling of biological flows including cardiovascular and respiratory systems, transport processes, and development of numerical tools for biomedical applications operated with patient-specific data. He is the author of more than 60 publications in these fields. With his colleagues, he developed a complex numerical model of respiratory and cardiovascular system with regulatory mechanisms, a method of numerical assessment of haemodynamic significance of the stenosis in coronary and cerebral vessels, a model of microcirculation during tumor angiogenesis, and a model of blood flow during intensive exercise.

Applications of Modeling and Machine Learning in Endurance Sports

Mikhail Vinogradov

Innovation center of Russian Olympic Committee, Moscow, Russia
vinogradov.coach@gmail.com

Abstract. Mathematical and computer models may provide a method of describing and predicting the effect of training on endurance performance. Various tools (statistical models, dose–response modeling, machine learning algorithms, critical power models) are employed in endurance sports. Current approaches have some advantages and limitations (especially in elite sports). Usually, training and performance data are used in these methods. But in order to increase the quality of the models such variables as recovery data, social-psychological stress data, altitude, and heat exposure data should be included.

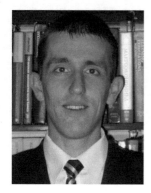

Bio. For the period 2000–2008, Mikhail A. Vinogradov worked as an assistant professor (Altai State University, Russia), 2008 to 2010: Associate Professor (Altai State University, Russia). In 2011–2012, Mikhail A. Vinogradov worked as a main coach in Halden Skiklubb (Norway). Mikhail A. Vinogradov has been working as a personal coach for several elite and World class O-athletes. His runners won all kinds of titles from biggest international O-relays (including World Championships). Mikhail A. Vinogradov worked with Russian National team (2010–2017). Nowadays, he is Ph.D., Lead Expert (Moscow Center of Advanced Sport Technologies) and Expert (Innovation center of Russian Olympic Committee). He was honored as coach of Russia (2018). Current science interests include modeling, data mining, and cognitive biases in sports.

Visual Analytics of Sports Data

Yingcai Wu

Zhejiang University, Hangzhou, Zhejiang, China
ycwu@zju.edu.cn

Abstract. With the rapid development of sensing technologies and wearable devices, large amounts of sports data have been acquired daily. The data usually imply a wide spectrum of information and rich knowledge about sports. However, extracting insights from the complex sports data has become more challenging for analysts using traditional automatic approaches, such as data mining and statistical analysis. Visual analytics is an emerging research area which aims to support "analytical reasoning facilitated by interactive visual interfaces." It has proven its value to tackle various important problems in sports science, such as tactics analysis in table tennis and formation analysis in soccer. Visual analytics would enable coaches and analysts to cope with complex sports data in an interactive and intuitive manner. In this talk, I will discuss our research experiences in visual analytics of sports data and introduce several recent studies of our group of making sense of sports data through interactive visualization.

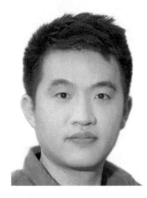

Bio. Yingcai Wu is a National Youth-1000 scholar and a ZJU100 Young Professor at the State Key Laboratory of CAD and CG, College of Computer Science and Technology, Zhejiang University. He obtained his Ph.D. degree in Computer Science from the Hong Kong University of Science and Technology (HKUST). Prior to his current position, Yingcai Wu was a researcher in Microsoft Research Asia, Beijing, China, from 2012 to 2015, and a postdoctoral researcher at the University of California, Davis, from 2010 to 2012. He was a paper co-chair of IEEE Pacific Visualization 2017, ChinaVis 2016, ChinaVis 2017, and VINCI 2014. He was also the guest editor of IEEE TVCG, ACM Transactions on Intelligent Systems and Technology (TIST), and IEEE Transactions on Multimedia.

Contents

Applications in Sports Analytics

Assessing the Performances
of Soccer Players

Jesse Davis[1]([✉]), Lotte Bransen[2], Tom Decroos[1], Pieter Robberechts[1],
and Jan Van Haaren[2]

[1] Department of Computer Science, KU Leuven, Leuven, Belgium
{jesse.davis,tom.decroos,pieter.robberechts}@cs.kuleuven.be
[2] SciSports, Amersfoort, The Netherlands
{l.bransen,j.vanhaaren}@scisports.com

Abstract. A key question within sports analytics is how to analyze match data in order to objectively assess a player's performance during a match. This paper summarizes our recent attempts to address this question for soccer. First, we look at how to assign a value to each on-the-ball action a soccer player performs during a match. Second, we explore how these values depend on the level of mental pressure that the player experienced when performing the action. We conclude by briefly highlighting some potential applications of this work.

Keywords: Soccer analytics · Rating actions in soccer · Performance under mental pressure

1 Introduction

Interest in the field of *sports analytics* has exploded over the past decade. This interest has been driven by teams successfully employing data-driven techniques[1] and fan interest in sports and statistics. The increased interest has been fueled by new data sources such as

- event stream data, which provides information such as the time and location of specific events during a match;
- tracking data, which records positional data for all players and the ball multiple times per second; and
- sensors for heart rate, accelerometer and GPS, which allow for continuously monitoring athletes during training and competition.

These data are commonly and widely collected across multiple different sports.

The volume, richness and complexity of these types of data has spurred interest in using techniques from machine learning and data mining to analyze them. People have performed data-driven analyses for a variety of team sports,

---

[1] http://www.espn.com/espn/feature/story/_/id/12331388/the-great-analytics-rankings.

© Springer Nature Switzerland AG 2020
M. Lames et al. (Eds.): IACSS 2019, AISC 1028, pp. 3–10, 2020.
https://doi.org/10.1007/978-3-030-35048-2_1

including basketball [18, 26], American football [9, 21], soccer [8, 22, 25], and volleyball [28] as well as individual sports such as running [19, 24], tennis [31], and speed skating [13]. One line of work focuses on analyzing technical performance data arising from matches to address issues such as evaluating and identifying various tactics employed by teams [2, 3, 16, 20, 27, 29]. Similarly, there is also interest in analyzing the continuous monitoring data arising from the athletes themselves in order to gain insight into how to best manage their training load and optimize performance [10, 11, 30].

One canonical sports analytics question for team sports is the following:

How can we objectively assess a player's performance during a match?

Researchers and fans have explored deriving metrics that provide insights into this question for several different sports, including ice hockey [15], basketball [4], and soccer [7, 14]. Typically, these metrics try to assign a numeric value to each action a player has performed. This problem is challenging for several reasons. First, many actions (e.g., passes) do not directly lead to a quantifiable event (i.e., a goal or basket) that directly affects the match result. This problem is particularly pronounced in sports like ice hockey and soccer where goals are very rare events. Second, often times approaches only have access to event stream or play-by-play data as optical tracking data is often not distributed publicly and is costly to obtain. This means that the only information available is about the player who possesses the ball during the play. Unfortunately, approaches based on this type of data cannot value off-the-ball movements, which are very important from a tactical perspective. Finally, the game context also could influence performance: a player may behave differently in a tight match as opposed to a blowout.

This paper serves as a companion to my invited talk at the symposium, which will tie together several lines of our research related to assessing a soccer player's performance based on event stream data [1, 6, 7]. First, I will discuss our approach [7] for assigning values to all on-the-ball actions performed during a match. Intuitively, our action values capture an action's expected contribution to the match's goal difference. Our approach goes beyond ideas like expected goals [17] or assists by considering 21 different types of actions such as passes, crosses, dribbles, take-ons, and shots. Second, I will discuss how to analyze whether a player's performance is affected by mental pressure. When measuring mental pressure, we consider both the match context and the current game state. We first train one model that predicts the pre-match pressure and another that measures the in-game pressure, and then combine their outputs to derive a pressure level for each moment of a match. To gain an insight into how performance varies with respect to pressure, we compare a player's performances (i.e., action values) across different levels of mental pressure.

2   Data

Two primary data sources about soccer matches exist: event stream data and optical tracking data. Event stream data annotates the times and locations of specific events (e.g., passes, shots, cards, etc.) that occur in a match. Optical tracking data records the locations of the players and the ball at a high frequency using optical tracking systems during matches. In this work, we use event stream data because it is more widely available, which allows us to include many more players and teams in our analysis.

3 Evaluating Actions in Soccer Matches

A fundamental task in soccer analytics is to understand the value of each action a player performs during a match. This task can be formally defined as follows:

Given: An on-the-ball action a_i in game state s_i;
Do: Learn a function that assigns a contribution rating $CR(a_i)$ to the action.

The effect of every on-the-ball action is that it alters the game state. Our approach to rating actions [7] is based on measuring how valuable this resulting change of game state is:

$$CR(s_i, a_i) = V(s_{i+1}) - V(s_i), \tag{1}$$

where $V(.)$ represents the value of a game state and s_{i+1} is the game state that results from executing action a_i in game state s_i. Hence, the primary question becomes: How should we value a game state?

Intuitively, a helpful action is one that benefits a player's team, either by increasing the chance that his team scores or decreasing the chance that the opposing team scores. These actions should be positively valued. In contrast, actions that do the opposite are hurting the player's team and should be negatively valued. That suggests that one way to value a game state s_i is:

$$V(s_i) = P^k_{score}(s_i) - P^k_{concede}(s_i), \tag{2}$$

where $P^k_{score}(s_i)$ $(P^k_{concede}(s_i))$ is the probability that the team possessing the ball in state s_i will score (concede) in the next k actions. Typically, k should be some small number like five or ten as the effects of most actions will be temporally limited. Practically, the task becomes estimating these two probabilities for each game state, which can be solved by training any machine learning model that predicts a probability.

As always, the key to achieving good performance has less to do with picking the right model class and more to do with constructing a reasonable set of features. Here, the features need to accurately describe the game state. Important features include characteristics of the action itself such as its location and type. Similarly, the current time and score differential are also relevant. Finally, it is important to capture aspects about the current tempo in the game. A good proxy for this is measuring how fast the ball is moving as represented by distance covered and time elapsed between consecutive actions.

4   Modeling Pressure

Our hypothesis is that two factors affect mental pressure:

1. the pre-game context such as whether it is a home game or if the opponent is a traditional rival; and
2. the in-game context such as the time remaining and the current goal difference.

Therefore, we model the total mental pressure [1] for a game g currently at game state s_i as:

$$MP(g, s_i) = Pressure_{pre-game}(g) \times Pressure_{in-game}(s_i). \tag{3}$$

Next, we describe how to compute each metric.

4.1   Pre-game Pressure

A number of factors will affect the mental pressure surrounding a match:

Game Context. The properties of a game such as its location (i.e., home or away) and whether the opponent is a rival will affect the pressure.

Recent Form. A run of bad results, particularly for large clubs, will result in elevated pressure.

Team Context. Larger and more prestigious clubs tend to face more scrutiny and hence more pressure.

Game Importance. Each team has goals for a season, such as winning the league or simply staying up, that affect its pre-game pressure level. How much a game will affect a team's chance to achieve its goals will affect the pressure level.

We describe each match by hand-crafting a number of features corresponding to each of the four aforementioned categories of factors that affect pre-game pressure (see [1] for more details).

Unfortunately, games are not labeled with categories such as low pressure, normal pressure or high pressure. While assigning a concrete pressure level to a match may be challenging for a human annotator, given two matches and their contexts, it is easier to assess which one has higher stakes. This suggests that it is possible to address this as a ranking problem and apply techniques from machine learning to learn a ranker that predicts the pre-game pressure level for each game. We used a panel of 19 soccer experts and obtained 330 pairwise rankings from a randomly selected set of 170 games from the 2016/2017 and 2017/2018 Premier League, Bundesliga and LaLiga seasons. Additionally, to validate our model, we obtained 483 pairwise ratings for a diverse set of 20 games, including some crucial relegation games, rivalries, games of teams underperforming and end-of-season games where nothing was at stake anymore. We used these pairwise rankings and learned a Gradient Boosted Ranking Trees model to predict the pre-game pressure.

An accurate model should come close to mimicking the experts' aggregate (partial) ordering of these matches' pressure levels. However, the experts may not rank each pair in the same way (i.e., there is no consensus ordering), so an accurate model should perform similarly to the inter-expert agreement. Our learned model achieved an agreement of 73.91% with the annotators' rankings, which is close to the inter-expert agreement of 79.79%.

4.2   In-Game Pressure

The mental pressure experienced by players will vary over the course of the game as it depends on the current game state. Intuitively, mental pressure should be higher when scoring a goal would have a large impact on achieving a favorable match outcome such as a tie game with little time remaining. Conversely, pressure should be low when a goal would have a minimal effect on the result. For example, if the home team is winning $3 - 0$, scoring another goal is not particularly helpful.[2] We capture these intuitions by employing a win probability model [23]. Specifically, we look at the difference in win probability between the current game state and two hypothetical game states where the home or away team has scored an additional goal.

Because soccer is a low-scoring game, we model the win probability by predicting the future number of goals each team will score between now and the end of the match. We predicted the number of goals that the home ($y_h > t$) and away ($y_a > t$) team will score after time t using independent Binomial distributions:

$$y_h > t \mid \Theta_{t,home} \sim B(T - t, \Theta_{t,h}), \qquad (4)$$
$$y_a > t \mid \Theta_{t,away} \sim B(T - t, \Theta_{t,a}), \qquad (5)$$

where the parameters represent each team's estimated scoring intensity in the tth time frame. We estimate these scoring intensities from the current game state. We represent the game state using features such as the goal difference, the number of goals scored by each team, and the time remaining in the game.

This model allows us to predict a distribution over the estimated number of goals each team will have scored at the end of the game. From these totals, we can derive a distribution over the win-draw-loss probabilities at each specific time point.

5   Applications

Rating actions and measuring mental pressure has a number of interesting applications within the context of soccer.

Rating Players. The most obvious use of our metric is to rate players. This can be done for different time windows such as a game or a season. Similarly, it is possible to rate a player's abilities for each action type. These ratings could be used to, e.g., construct a team of the season. Similarly, they may be of interest to fans who are debating which player is better.

---

[2] Ignoring issues like overall goal difference as a tie breaker.

Identifying Match Highlights. One interesting problem within the context of sports is attempting to identify highlights within a match (c.f. [5,12]). This could be useful for a variety of end-users, such as fans who want to pick a selection of clips to watch, journalists who are tasked with writing a match report, or for a "highlight channel", which shows live action from multiple matches based on which match is currently the most interesting to follow. Potentially interesting events in a match could be identified by either (1) looking at high-pressure time periods or (2) considering both highly- and lowly-rated (because they represent a missed chance) actions.

Scouting for Player Acquisition. Looking at a player's performance ratings for various action types and in various game contexts could be a piece of information that scouting directors consider when searching for new players. For example, Leicester City signed Rachid Ghezzal as a replacement for Riyad Marhez in the summer of 2018. Xherdan Shaqiri also moved clubs in the summer of 2018 for a slightly higher transfer fee. Our analyses show that he may have been a better fit in terms of replicating Marhez's skills, particularly in terms of performing under pressure [1].

Performing Tactical Analyses. Player ratings and understanding performance under mental pressure can help inform decisions in three important ways. First, it could play a role in selecting a lineup or making a substitution. For example, we have found that some players (e.g., Alvaro Morata [1]) do not perform well under pressure, and hence may be less suitable for selection or candidates to be subbed off in such situations. Second, it can help evaluate different tactics. We have found that teams treat throw-ins differently between low-pressure and high-pressure situations [1]. For almost all teams, the contribution rating for throw-ins is higher in high-pressure situations than low-pressure ones. This is an interesting observation which suggests that teams miss the opportunity to create more danger with throw-ins early in the game. Finally, it could be used to gain an understanding of an opposing player's strengthens and weaknesses. For example, Harry Kane does not generate much value with his crosses [7].

6   Conclusions

This paper summarized our recent work on objectively assessing the performance of soccer players in various contexts based on event-stream data. This is a problem in sports analytics that has many use-cases such as rating players, scouting, highlight detection, and tactical analysis among others.

Acknowledgements. Jesse Davis is partially supported by the EU Interreg VA project Nano4Sports and the KU Leuven Research Fund (C14/17/07, C32/17/036). Tom Decroos is supported by Research Foundation-Flanders (FWO-Vlaanderen). Pieter Robberechts is supported by the EU Interreg VA project Nano4Sports.

References

1. Bransen, L., Robberechts, P., Van Haaren, J., Davis, J.: Choke or shine? Quantifying soccer players' abilities to perform under mental pressure. In: MIT Sloan Sports Analytics Conference (2019)
2. Bransen, L., Van Haaren, J., van de Velden, M.: Measuring soccer players' contributions to chance creation by valuing their passes. J. Quant. Anal. Sport. **15**, 97–116 (2019)
3. Brefeld, U., Lasek, J., Mair, S.: Probabilistic movement models and zones of control. Mach. Learn. **108**(1), 127–147 (2018)
4. Cervone, D., D'Amour, A., Bornn, L., Goldsberry, K.: POINTWISE: predicting points and valuing decisions in real time with NBA optical tracking data. In: MIT Sloan Sports Analytics Conference (2014)
5. Decroos, T., Dzyuba, V., Van Haaren, J., Davis, J.: Predicting soccer highlights from spatio-temporal match event streams. In: Proceedings of the Thirty-First AAAI Conference on Artificial Intelligence, pp. 1302–1308 (2017)
6. Decroos, T., Van Haaren, J., Dzyuba, V., Davis, J.: STARSS: a spatio-temporal action rating system for soccer. In: Proceedings of the Fourth Workshop on Machine Learning and Data Mining for Sports Analytics, pp. 11–20 (2017)
7. Decroos, T., Bransen, L., Van Haaren, J., Davis, J.: Actions speak louder than goals: valuing player actions in soccer. In: Proceedings of the 25th ACM SIGKDD International Conference on Knowledge Discovery & Data Mining, pp. 1851–1861 (2019)
8. Decroos, T., Van Haaren, J., Davis, J.: Automatic discovery of tactics in spatio-temporal soccer match data. In: Proceedings of the 24th ACM SIGKDD International Conference on Knowledge Discovery & Data Mining, pp. 223–232 (2018)
9. Goldner, K.: A Markov model of football: using stochastic processes to model a football drive. J. Quant. Anal. Sport. **8**(1), (2012)
10. Jaspers, A., Op De Beéck, T., Brink, M.S., Frencken, W.G., Staes, F., Davis, J.J., Helsen, W.F.: Relationships between the external and internal training load in professional soccer: what can we learn from machine learning? Int. J. Sport. Physiol. Perform. **13**(5), 625–630 (2018)
11. Jaspers, A., Op De Beéck, T., Brink, M.S., Frencken, W.G., Staes, F., Davis, J., Helsen, W.: Predicting future perceived wellness in professional soccer: the role of preceding load and wellness. Int. J. Sport. Physiol. Perform. **14**(8), 1074–1080 (2019)
12. Keane, E., Desaulniers, P., Bornn, L., Javan, M.: Data-driven lowlight and highlight reel creation based on explainable temporal game models. In: MIT Sloan Sports Analytics Conference (2019)
13. Knobbe, A.J., Orie, J., Hofman, N., van der Burgh, B., Cachucho, R.: Sports analytics for professional speed skating. Data Min. Knowl. Discov. **31**(6), 1872–1902 (2017)
14. Link, D., Lang, S., Seidenschwarz, P.: Real time quantification of dangerousity in football using spatiotemporal tracking data. PLoS ONE **11**(12), e0168768 (2016)
15. Liu, G., Schulte, O.: Deep reinforcement learning in ice hockey for context-aware player evaluation. In: Proceedings of the Twenty-Seventh International Joint Conference on Artificial Intelligence, pp. 3442–3448 (2018)
16. Lucey, P., Oliver, D., Carr, P., Roth, J., Matthews, I.: Assessing team strategy using spatiotemporal data. In: Proceedings of the 19th International Conference on Knowledge Discovery and Data Mining, pp. 1366–1374 (2013)

17. Lucey, P, Monfort, M., Bialkowski, A., Carr, P., Matthews, I.: Quality vs quantity: improved shot prediction in soccer using strategic features from spatiotemporal data. In: MIT Sloan Sports Analytics Conference (2015)
18. Miller, A.C., Bornn, L., Adams, R.P., Goldsberry, K.: Factorized point process intensities: a spatial analysis of professional basketball. In: Proceedings of the 31th International Conference on Machine Learning, pp. 235–243 (2014)
19. Op De Beéck, T., Meert, W., Schütte, K., Vanwanseele, B., Davis, J.: Fatigue prediction in outdoor runners via machine learning and sensor fusion. In: Proceedings of the 24th ACM SIGKDD International Conference on Knowledge Discovery & Data Mining, pp. 606–615 (2018)
20. Pappalardo, L., Cintia, P., Ferragina, P., Massucco, E., Pedreschi, D., Giannotti, F.: PlayeRank: multi-dimensional and role-aware rating of soccer player performance. CoRR abs/1802.04987 (2018)
21. Pelechrinis, K., Papalexakis, E.: The anatomy of american football: evidence from 7 years of NFL game data. PLoS ONE **11**(12), e0168716 (2018)
22. Rein, R., Raabe, D., Perl, J., Memmert, D.: Evaluation of changes in space control due to passing behavior in elite soccer using Voronoi-cells. In: Proceedings of the 10th International Symposium on Computer Science in Sports, pp. 179–183 (2016)
23. Robberechts, P., Van Haaren, J., Davis, J.: Who will win it? An in-game win probability model for football. arXiv:1906.05029 (2019)
24. Smyth, B., Cunningham, P.: Marathon race planning: a case-based reasoning approach. In: Proceedings of the Twenty-Seventh International Joint Conference on Artificial Intelligence, pp. 5364–5368 (2018)
25. Spearman, W.: Beyond expected goals. In: MIT Sloan Sports Analytics Conference (2018)
26. van Bommel, M., Bornn, L.: Adjusting for scorekeeper bias in NBA box scores. Data Min. Knowl. Discov. **31**(6), 1622–1642 (2017)
27. Van Haaren, J., Dzyuba, V., Hannosset, S., Davis, J.: Automatically discovering offensive patterns in soccer match data. In: Advances in Intelligent Data Analysis XIV, pp. 286–297 (2015)
28. Van Haaren, J., Ben Shitrit, H., Davis, J., Fua, P.: Analyzing volleyball match data from the 2014 world championships using machine learning techniques. In: Proceedings of the 22nd ACM SIGKDD International Conference on Knowledge Discovery and Data Mining. ACM, pp. 627–634 (2016)
29. Van Haaren, J., Hannosset, S., Davis, J.: Strategy discovery in professional soccer match data. In: Proceedings of the KDD-16 Workshop on Large-Scale Sports Analytics, pp. 1–4 (2016)
30. Vandewiele, G., Geurkink, Y., Lievens, M., Ongenae, F., Turck, F.D., Boone, J.: Enabling training personalization by predicting the sessioon rate of perceived exertion. In: Proceedings of the Machine Learning and Data Mining for Sports Analytics ECML/PKDD 2018 Workshop (2017)
31. Wei, X., Lucey, P., Morgan, S., Sridharan, S.: Forecasting the next shot location in tennis using fine-grained spatiotemporal tracking data. IEEE Trans. Knowl. Data Eng. **28**(11), 2988–2997 (2016)

Fitting Motion Models to Contextual Player Behavior

Bartholomew Spencer[1]([⊠]) [ID], Karl Jackson[2] [ID],
and Sam Robertson[1] [ID]

[1] Institute for Health and Sport (IHeS),
Victoria University, Melbourne, Australia
bartholomew.spencer@vu.edu.au
[2] Champion Data Pty Ltd., Melbourne, Australia

Abstract. The objective of this study was to incorporate contextual information into the modelling of player movements. This was achieved by combining the distributions of forthcoming passing contests that players committed to and those they did not. The resultant array measures the probability a player would commit to forthcoming contests in their vicinity. Commitment-based motion models were fit on 46220 samples of player behavior in the Australian Football League. It was found that the shape of commitment-based models differed greatly to displacement-based models for Australian footballers. Player commitment arrays were used to measure the spatial occupancy and dominance of the attacking team. The spatial characteristics of pass receivers were extracted for 2934 passes. Positional trends in passing were identified. Furthermore, passes were clustered into three components using Gaussian mixture models. Passes in the AFL are most commonly to one-on-one contests or unmarked players. Furthermore, passes were rarely greater than 25 m.

Keywords: Player motion · Spatiotemporal · Australian football

1 Introduction

The measurement of a player's spatial occupancy can reveal insights into space, congestion and passing opportunities. While early research into spatial occupancy considered players as fixed objects, recent iterations of Voronoi-like dominant regions have incorporated the effects of player motion [1, 2]. Underlying these approaches is limited consideration of the continuous nature of space. Should the application of spatial occupancy involve possession outcomes, space should be considered relative to the ball.

Recent studies have addressed this concept. Fernandez and Bornn [3] measured the spatial dominance of teams by representing a player's influence as a bivariate normal distribution. The result considers the continuous nature of space but is not fit on empirical data. Brefeld [2] fit player motion models on the distribution of a player's observed displacements but did not consider the context of those displacements (i.e., the current possession location). Logically, the amount of spatial dominance a team exhibits over a location need be measured relative to how players would control said space if the ball were moved to that location.

© Springer Nature Switzerland AG 2020
M. Lames et al. (Eds.): IACSS 2019, AISC 1028, pp. 11–18, 2020.
https://doi.org/10.1007/978-3-030-35048-2_2

In this study we present a method of fitting player motion models with consideration of displacement context. Models are fit on player commitment to passing contests, rather than raw displacements. Resultant models measure the probability a player would contest a pass to locations in their vicinity. We demonstrate the applications of these models in the analysis of kicking in the Australian Football League (AFL).

2 Methods

Ball tracking is not commercially available in AFL; however, ball location can be inferred from play-by-play data. Player motion models are proposed as an adequate forecast of future behaviours in the absence of precision ball tracking. Hence, the objective of this study was to model player motion with consideration of the context of player displacements, without increasing their dimensionality beyond consideration of location, velocity and time.

2.1 Data and Pre-processing

LPS player-tracking data (x, y, t) were collected from the 2017 and 2018 AFL seasons. Tracking data (10 Hz) were consolidated with play-by-play event data (known as transactions). Transactions are recorded to the nearest second, hence are assumed to occur at the beginning of the second when combined with LPS datasets. Player orientation and velocity were calculated from the tracking data under the assumption that players were oriented in the direction of their movement. For analysis, passes that begin with and ended with a mark were extracted (*mark-to-mark* passes). This constraint ensured that location could be inferred. A *mark* is awarded when a) a player catches a kick on the full, and b) the kick travelled at minimum of 15 m.

2.2 Possession Contests

Commitment models are fit on player participation to forthcoming passing contests. Passing contests are pass events in which more than one player attempts to win the ball. In the AFL datasets, events that fit this criterion are *contested marks* and *spoils* transactions. The former refers to a pass caught by a player while under pressure and the latter relates to a marking attempt in which the ball is knocked away by an opponent. Passing contests are henceforth referred to as contests.

2.3 Modelling Process

Each contest involves two events of interest: the pass that preceded the contest and the contest transaction. The timestamps of these events are referred to as t_p and t_c respectively. When referring to a player's commitment we are referring to the likelihood a player will commit to a forthcoming contest, given their position and momentum at t_p. The commitment modelling process is as follows:

1. Player momentum and position at t_p and the ball's travel time, or *time-to-point*, are recorded. The latter is simply $t_c - t_p$.

2. For each player, compute the relative location of the contest. This relative location is considered a potential player displacement. The relative location is as follows:

$$\theta = cos^{-1}\left(\frac{\vec{AB} \cdot \vec{BC}}{\left\|\vec{AB}\right\| \cdot \left\|\vec{BC}\right\|}\right) \tag{1}$$

$$(x, y) = (d \cdot \cos \theta, d \cdot \sin \theta) \tag{2}$$

where AB is the player's movement vector, BC is the displacement vector to the contest and d is the Euclidean distance between the player and the contest.

3. If the Euclidean distance between the player and the contest is less than two meters at t_c, player commitment (C) is recorded as 1 (hence, the player realized the potential displacement), else if greater than two meters, commitment is recorded as 0.
4. The dataset is partitioned into *commitment* and *no commitment* sets along C.
5. Distribution of both datasets is estimated via Kernel density estimation (KDE) with Gaussian kernels. Datasets are four-dimensional, containing the relative contest location (x, y), player velocity (v) and ball time-to-point (t).
6. The distributions are combined, weighted according to event frequency, using the following function:

$$p_i(x, y, v, t) = \frac{wf_{C=1}(x, y, v, t)}{wf_{C=1}(x, y, v, t) + (1 - w)f_{C=0}(x, y, v, t)} \tag{3}$$

where $f_{C=1}$ and $f_{C=0}$ are the distributions, and w is the weight.

The two-meter threshold for player commitment (step 3) was chosen as an adequate distance after discussion with AFL analysts. Individual distributions represent the density of contests that were committed to ($f_{C=1}$) and those that were ignored ($f_{C=0}$). By combining the distributions (Eq. 3) the resulting variable (p_i) measures the probability that a new sample (given x, y, v, t) belongs to the commitment distribution. The resultant array measures a player's spatial influence. A player's influence is a forecast of their behaviors in respect to a forthcoming passing contest.

2.4   Spatial Metrics

We measure the spatial influence of a team as the sum of the influence of its players:

$$Inf(x, y) = \sum_{i=1}^{18} Pr_i \tag{4}$$

and dominance is the proportion of space a team owns at a location:

$$Dom_a(x, y) = \frac{Inf_a(x, y)}{Inf_a(x, y) + Inf_o(x, y)} \tag{5}$$

2.5 Passing Analysis

Commitment models are used to analyse characteristics of passes. Mark-to-mark passes were extracted from the transactional dataset. The kicking distance (metres), spatial dominance, influence and *equity* of passes were recorded. AFL field equity (FE) is a measure of the value of space described in [4]. The equity of a pass is the change in FE between the passer and receiver ($equity = FE_{receiver} - FE_{passer}$). Metrics were analyzed at different field locations. Spearman correlation coefficient was used to assess the relationship between metrics and the distance between the receiver and the attacking goals. To define passing types, characteristics of passes were clustered via Gaussian mixture models, with the number of components chosen via the elbow method [5].

3 Results

An example output visualizing the spatial dominance and influence of an attacking team is presented in Fig. 1, where areas of darker green represent higher dominance.

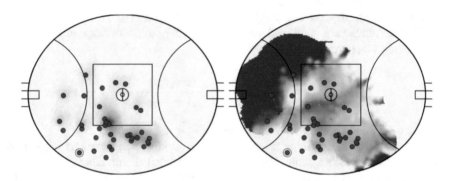

Fig. 1. Example output of spatial influence (left) and dominance (right) for the attacking team (in blue). The player with possession is circled in yellow (towards the lower boundary). The attacking team is moving from left to right. Spatial influence is the sum of player commitment models across a team (see Eq. 4) and dominance is a measure of spatial control derived from both team's influence (see Eq. 5). Darker green areas indicate higher values for the attacking team.

3.1 Commitment Models

Player commitment behavior was recorded for 46220 samples. The $C = 1$ and $C = 0$ datasets consisted of 6392 and 39828 samples ($w = 0.14$). Figure 2 visualizes commitment models for two velocities for $t = 2$ s. These are compared to motion models fit on player displacements (as in [2]). Fitting displacements (Fig. 2b, d) suggests players are unlikely to reorient, hence are insufficient for modelling behavior to forthcoming contests.

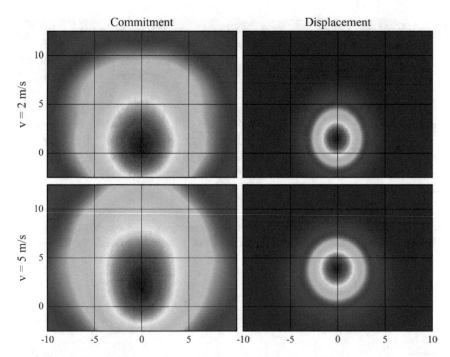

Fig. 2. Player commitment (left) and displacement (right) motion models for $v = 2$ m/s (top) and $v = 5$ m/s (bottom). Density represents the probability of making a displacement.

3.2   Passing Analysis

A total of 2934 passes were analyzed. Two-dimensional distributions of passing features are presented in Fig. 3. Dominance of passes is bimodal. The dominance and influence of receivers was recorded and smoothed by field location (Fig. 4). There is a trend towards passes to lower dominance receivers towards the attacking goal. Furthermore, influence of receivers is high in the forward 50 region. This is indicative of kicks to congested groups, rather than individual players. Minimal correlation was found between the distance to objective and both dominance ($\rho = 0.05$, $p < 0.01$) and influence ($\rho = -0.08$, $p < 0.01$).

3.3   Passing Clusters

Passes were clustered via GMM into three components. Component means are visualized in two-dimensions in Fig. 3. Characteristics of the components are presented in Table 1. Component 1 represents a medium-range pass to a group of players in congestion (*influence* > 0.5, *dominance* < 1.0), component 2 is a short-range pass to an open player (*dominance* = 1.0) and component 3 is a short-range pass to a one-on-one contest (*influence* < 0.5, *dominance* < 1.0).

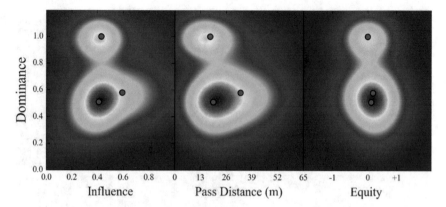

Fig. 3. Distributions (estimated via KDE) of (a) Influence, (b) Distance and (c) Equity relative to Dominance. GMM Component means are presented as magenta points in the 2D plots.

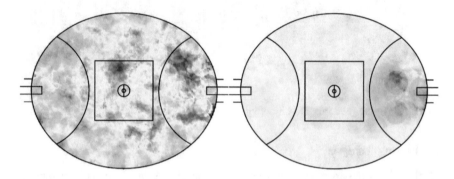

Fig. 4. Smoothed spatial dominance (left) and influence (right) of pass receivers. Attacking team is moving left to right. High dominance and influence is indicated by darker green regions.

Table 1. The weight and means of Gaussian mixture model components.

Variable	Component 1	Component 2	Component 3
Weight	0.43	0.24	0.33
Dominance (%)	0.58	1.00	0.51
Influence	0.59	0.43	0.41
Distance (m)	33.3	17.9	19.4
Equity	0.09	0.00	0.06

4   Discussion

This study presented a method for fitting player motion models with consideration of the context of player displacements. This was achieved via the fitting of participation to forthcoming events, rather than to observed player displacements, representing a new approach to player motion models. Additionally, the models in this study fit the distribution of samples in four-dimensions, choosing to consider velocity and time as continuous rather than categorical as in [2].

It was observed that commitment models suggest a higher likelihood of reorientation than motion models fit on player displacements (see Fig. 2). In particular, displacement-based models forecast very few repositions in the negative y- axis. Observation of player commitment behaviors suggest reorientation is possible in all directions. The low probability of reorientation in displacement-based motion models is likely due to the nature of gameplay in AFL. The large field size and typical gameplay result in players frequently following the ball, rather than holding formations. Hence, for the analysis demonstrated in this study, motion models fit on player displacements are inadequate for describing future behavior.

Commitment models are fit on behavior to the next possession, hence are limited to applications that consider short-term behavior. At higher velocities, the spread of a player's influence increases and the shape changes (see Fig. 2). These considerations do not affect the applications presented in this study. It should be noted that commitment models were fit on 46220 samples which is roughly equivalent to the number of one-second displacements a player would make in a single match. As a result, these models may be less smooth than motion models fit on displacements (Fig. 2). Bandwidth selection during the fitting process can be modified to account for this.

A noteworthy limitation of commitment models is a reliance on transactions of differing frequency to player-tracking datasets. As a result, transactions and player-tracking may be misaligned by up to one second. The generous commitment radius of two metres deals with this to an extent, however higher frequency transactions would reduce the noise of resultant models.

Studies analyzing passing in the AFL have previously utilized discrete passing features and manually collected data (e.g., [6]). The computation of spatial features presents continuous metrics for passing analysis. Spatial dominance of receivers was found to be bimodal at dominance of an equal contest (dominance = 0.5) and an open player (dominance = 1.0). It was noted that passes to open players were rarely greater than 25 m. There is an indication that the spatial characteristics of receivers differs by region, despite minimal correlation between these metrics and a player's distance to the goalposts. In particular, the influence of receivers was higher in the forward 50 region than elsewhere. This is indicative of a pass to a congested group of players. Furthermore, early results show that receiver dominance is higher in the defensive 50 region, indicative of risk aversion in defensive positions. These results may be explained by team formations. Players have more space to work with when a team has possession in their defensive 50. This space decreases as the ball is moved towards the attacking goalposts, hence players become more congested.

Analysis of the spatial characteristics of passing produced three passing clusters. While the equity of all components was minimal, the short-range pass to an open player (component 2) had a mean equity of 0.00, hence does not typically improved a team's scoring chance. This may be a pass to stall play in the absence of better options. The low mean passing distance of components 2 and 3 (< 20 m) suggests a tendency to execute short-range passes.

While the analysis in this study has focused on on-ball possessions, measures of spatial occupancy have applications in off-ball analysis. Fernandez and Bornn [3] utilized similar methodology to analyze space creation of off-ball actions in soccer. Future applications of spatial occupancy should continue the development of these topics.

5 Conclusion

A new method for measuring player spatial occupancy was exemplified in this study. The occupancy of Australian footballers was estimated via the probability they would reposition to forthcoming passes contests. When compared to displacement-based motion models in Australian football, commitment models were found to be a better representation of contextual player behavior. Resultant commitment models were used to describe the kicking landscape of AFL footballers, finding that passes were frequently to one-on-one contests or open players. Furthermore, long kicks are infrequent and there is a significance number of passes around the minimum marking distance.

References

1. Gudmundsson, J., Horton, M.: Spatio-temporal analysis of team sports. ACM Comput. Surv. **50**(2), 22 (2017). https://doi.org/10.1145/3054132
2. Brefeld, U., Lasek, J., Mair, S.: Probabilistic movement models and zones of control. Mach. Learn. **108**(1), 127–147 (2018). https://doi.org/10.1007/s10994-018-5725-1
3. Fernandez, J., Bornn, L.: Wide open spaces: a statistical technique for measuring space creation in professional soccer. In: Sloan Sports Analytics Conference (2018)
4. Jackson, K.: Assessing player performance in Australian football using spatial data. Doctoral dissertation, Ph.D. thesis, Swinburne University of Technology (2016)
5. Soni Madhulatha, T.: An overview of clustering methods. IOSR J. Eng. **2**(4), 719–725 (2012)
6. Robertson, S., Spencer, B., Back, N., Farrow, D.: A rule induction framework for the determination of representative learning design in skilled performance. J. Sport. Sci. 1–6 (2019). https://doi.org/10.1080/02640414.2018.1555905

A Flexible Approach to Football Analytics: Assessment, Modeling and Implementation

Philipp Seidenschwarz[1,2(✉)], Martin Rumo[1], Lukas Probst[2],
and Heiko Schuldt[2]

[1] Centre of Technologies in Sports and Medicine, Bern University
of Applied Sciences, Aarbergstrasse 5, 2560 Nidau-Biel, Switzerland
{philipp.seidenschwarz,martin.rumo}@bfh.ch
[2] Department of Mathematics and Computer Science, University of Basel,
Spiegelgasse 1, 4051 Basel, Switzerland
{philipp.seidenschwarz,lukas.probst,heiko.schuldt}@unibas.ch

Abstract. Quantitative analysis in football is difficult due to the complexity and continuous fluidity of the game. Even though there is an increased accessibility of spatio-temporal data, scientific approaches to extract valuable information are seldomly useful in practice. We propose a new approach to building an information system for football. This approach consists of a method to extract football-specific concepts from interviews, to formalize them in a performance model, and to define and implement the data structures and algorithms in STREAMTEAM, a framework for the detection of complex (team) events. In this paper we present this approach in detail and provide an example for its use.

Keywords: Football · Modeling · Event detection · Spatio-temporal data

1 Introduction

Over the past years, football has seen a steep increase in the availability of spatio-temporal data coming either from dedicated sensor systems or camera deployments. This development has given rise to novel types of questions analysts can ask [12]. Quantitative analysis in football is difficult due to the complexity and continuous fluidity of the game [3]. Yet, existing approaches aim at measuring high-level concepts in football such as individual and team ball possession [6] or pressure [1]. Nevertheless, it has been argued that the questions addressed by sport scientists often have small influence on football practice [2,7]. Off-ball performance, for example, is seldomly represented in match statistics. This is why coaches still heavily rely on time-consuming qualitative video analysis [4]. In order to make data useful for coaches, a system is needed that can extract information representing the coaches' concepts from spatio-temporal data.

© Springer Nature Switzerland AG 2020
M. Lames et al. (Eds.): IACSS 2019, AISC 1028, pp. 19–27, 2020.
https://doi.org/10.1007/978-3-030-35048-2_3

The coaching staff uses specific concepts when defining a match plan. The match plan represents a collection of tactical decisions that have been taken before a match. We will use the match plan to demonstrate our approach. Specific data objects and their implementation will be described by an example.

2 Approach

Our approach consists of extracting football-specific concepts from interviews and formalizing them in a performance model. This performance model is translated into a data model needed for subsequent implementation (see Fig. 1).

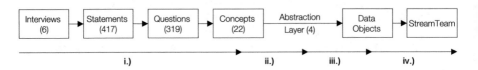

Fig. 1. Schematic representation of our approach: (i) performance factors assessment, (ii) performance modeling, (iii) data modeling, and (iv) system implementation

2.1 Performance Factors Assessment

To assess the coaches' way of analyzing, interpreting, and preparing a football match, semi-structured interviews were conducted. Only coaches $(n = 6)$ with an active UEFA Pro Licence are considered for the interview process. Questions are separated into nine different topics (see Table 1) and mainly relate to the information coaches take into account for the creation of their match plan.

Table 1. The nine topics of the interview guideline with sample questions and the number of resulting statements and questions of coaches (#)

Topic	Example question	#
Principles	What are possible reasons for changing the system?	97
Player Profiles	What are possible weaknesses of a player?	63
Offensive Organization	Where and how can the offense be started?	42
Opponent Information	How is an opponents' key player characterized?	41
Set Plays	How should the defense act in a corner kick situation?	26
Defensive Organization	How can the defense be organized?	24
Transition DEF-OFF	What options exist during transition DEF-OFF?	12
Build-up Play	What options exist during build-up play?	7
Transition OFF-DEF	What options exist during transition OFF-DEF?	7
Total		*319*

Interviews are recorded and transcribed. In a first step, examples and descriptions of specific situations are deleted and only general statements on concepts, patterns of play and arising questions are considered (n = 417). In a next step, these statements and questions are categorized into main categories and sub-categories following Kuckartz' approach of content-related structured qualitative analysis [5]. Only statements (n = 260) and questions (n = 59) that can be assigned to one of the nine topics of Table 1 are kept back for further processing. For each of the statements, a corresponding question is created that represents the coaches' need for information when setting up a match plan or adjusting it during the match. This step leads to a total number of 319 questions. In a next step, the underlying concepts are extracted for each of these questions. The example in Table 2 illustrates this procedure.

Table 2. Example for the extraction of concepts from coaches' statements

Step	Example
1. Statement	The defending team decides where to start a pressure situation
2. Question	Where does the defending team start a pressure situation?
3. Concept	Pressure

At this point of analysis we identify 22 football-specific concepts. These concepts and the corresponding number of questions are listed in Table 3.

Table 3. The 22 concepts with short description and number of questions (#)

Concept	Short description	#
Individuality	Player profile: mental, physical, tactical, technical	50
Line-up	Formation of a team and system of play	42
Attacking Play	Team speeds up, attempt to create a scoring opportunity	34
Pressure	Pressure of the defensive team on the offensive team	33
Principle	General idea how to play, line-up and movements	29
Running Trajectory	Trajectory per player from acceleration to deceleration	18
Coordination	Degree of team organization: compactness, synchronicity	14
Set Play Variation	Different options in offensive set plays	14
Defensive Play	Defensive schema after loss of ball possession	11
Cooperation	Profile of functional units: duos, trios, etc	9
Zonal Marking	Defending player covers a specific space on the pitch	9
Open Space	Open spaces on the pitch for the offensive team	8
Build-up Play	Before attacking play, intention to gain territory	7
Manipulating Space	Creating, defending, and using space on the pitch	7
Man-to-Man Marking	Assignment of a player to a direct opponent	7
Gain Possession	Player gains possession of the ball	6
Change of Speed	Transition from build-up play to attacking play	5
Duel	Two players involved, intention to gain/defend possession	5
Passing Option	Number of players with high likelihood to receive a pass	4
Lose Possession	Player loses possession of the ball	3
Fall Back	Defending players quickly getting behind the ball	2
Orientation	Orientation of a player relating to the opponents' goal	2
Total		*319*

2.2   Performance Modeling

In the performance modeling stage, the concepts are assigned to one of four abstraction layers: (i) atomic events, (ii) phases, (iii) continuous states, and (iv) profiles (see Fig. 2).

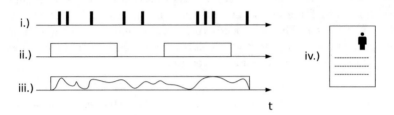

Fig. 2. The four layers of abstraction: (i) atomic events, (ii) phases, (iii) continuous states, and (iv) profiles

While the first three layers are descriptions of the dynamics of a match, profiles contain information that has been aggregated over a defined number of past matches.

Atomic Events. An atomic event is a distinct, basic and inseparable event that occurs at a specific time and that is characterized by an observable pattern. *Change of Speed, Duel, Gain Possession*, and *Lose Possession* are examples for such atomic events. Furthermore, atomic events can serve to segment the match into phases.

Phases. A phase segments the dynamics of the match. It has a beginning and an end. In a phase, information is aggregated over the time period delimited by the phase (e.g., number of passes during build-up play). The following concepts can be assigned to phases: *Attacking Play, Build-up Play, Defensive Play*, and *Set Play Variation*.

	Lose Possession	Gain Possession	Change of Speed	Duel	
...	**Defensive Play**	**Build-up Play**	**Attacking Play**	**Set Play Variation**	...
...	Fall Back	Passing Option		Man-to-Man Marking	...
...	Pressure	Manipulating Space		Zonal Marking	...
...		Running Trajectory			...
...	...	...		...	...

Fig. 3. Relation of atomic events, phases, and continuous states with highlighted *Defensive Play* stack used as an example for the data modeling and implementation stages

Continuous States. A continuous state is defined during a phase and further characterizes the latter. It denotes the evolution of a set of parameters over time. These parameters can be discrete (e.g., the number of players behind the ball) or continuous (e.g., the average distance between players). A continuous state can be defined for individual players (e.g., *Orientation, Running Trajectory*), for groups of players (e.g., *Coordination, Man-to-Man Marking, Zonal Marking*), or the entire team (e.g., *Fall Back, Manipulating Space, Open Space, Passing Option, Pressure*). While *Pressure* and *Fall Back* characterize a teams' *Defensive Play* phase, information about *Man-to-Man Marking* and *Zonal Marking* are specially important during defensive set play phases (see Fig. 3).

Profiles. A profile characterizes individual players, groups of players, or teams through aggregated information from previous matches. Individual player profiles may contain information on *Individuality*, for instance the physical fitness and summarized information on typical running trajectories. Profiles of groups of players (e.g., duos, trios, defensive line) may contain measures of *Cooperation*. Team profiles might contain typical *Line-ups* and *Principles*.

2.3   Data Modeling

In the data modeling stage, the performance model is translated into a data model which is needed for subsequent implementation. The data model consists of data objects with mandatory and optional attributes.

Atomic events have the following mandatory attributes: time-stamp, type, (x, y) coordinates, and references to the players involved. Optionally, one can add a set of qualifiers. The mandatory attributes for phases are their type and the references to the atomic events that delimit them. Optional attributes for phases are made up of information aggregated over the phase. Continuous states represent a metric evolving over time. It consists of a continuous stream of two mandatory attributes: a time stamp, and a metric (e.g., (x, y) coordinates of a running trajectory). Optional attributes can be used for meta data to further describe the metric (e.g., player reference to which the running trajectory is assigned). Profiles consist of one mandatory attribute, namely a reference to a player or a set of players. Optionally, a set of attributes that represent aggregated information from matches can be added to the profile.

The *Defensive Play* stack (see Fig. 3) can now be represented by five data objects. Two atomic events, namely *Lose Possession* and *Gain Possession*, that delimit the *Defensive Play* phase and two continuous states that add two evolving metrics to the description of the phase: a pressure index (*Pressure*), and the number of players behind the ball (*Fall Back*).

2.4   System Implementation in StreamTeam

In order to populate the data model with data from actual matches, an analysis system which detects patterns in position data streams and outputs the data objects described in Sect. 2.3 is needed. In our previous work, we have designed and implemented STREAMTEAM [10], a novel middleware for developing such team collaboration analysis systems. STREAMTEAM is based on Apache Samza [8], a generic data stream processing system. An analysis system based on the STREAMTEAM middleware is composed of workers which are combined to an analysis workflow. Each of these workers performs a part of the overall analysis task. This enables distributing the workload onto multiple machines and thus facilitates performing very comprehensive analyses in real-time.

STREAMTEAM-FOOTBALL, our football analysis system prototype presented in [11], is able to detect a multitude of different atomic events and phases, and to generate various continuous states. This is done on the basis of the raw positions of the players and the ball, which it consumes as elements of an input data stream. The detection is done in a workflow consisting of 13 parameterizable workers. This enables performance analysts to setup and configure their own STREAMTEAM-FOOTBALL deployment without changing a single line of code.

The current version of STREAMTEAM-FOOTBALL already provides implementations for the majority of the *Defensive Play* stack of the data model presented in Sect. 2.3. This includes a *Ball Possession Worker* which detects ball possession change events and thus *Gain Possession* and *Lose Possession* events by means of analyzing directional changes as well as velocity changes of the ball and the positions of the players. This worker consumes a positions stream which comprises elements shipping the current position of players and the ball, an auxiliary team sides stream (emitted by a *Kickoff Detection Worker*) whose elements specify the playing direction of each team, and an auxiliary ball in field stream (emitted by an *Area Detection Worker*) whose elements specify whether the ball is inside the field or not. Detected ball possession change events are emitted as elements of a ball possession change event stream. The schema of this stream together with a sample element is given in Table 4. These events mark the start and the end of a *Defensive Play* phase. In addition, STREAMTEAM-FOOTBALL provides a *Pressing Analysis Worker* which calculates the *Pressure* on the basis of this ball possession change event stream and the positions stream. This worker periodically emits a pressing index as an element of a pressing state stream.

It would be easily possible to add an additional *Defensive Play Phase Worker* which consumes the ball possession change event stream and actually emits data stream elements representing *Defensive Play* phases if this is required. Moreover, to implement the remainder of the *Defensive Play* stack, we could further add an additional *Fall Back Worker*. This worker could consume the ball possession change event stream to identify the team which is currently in possession of the ball and thus offensive, the auxiliary team sides stream to determine the playing direction of this team, and the positions stream to obtain the current positions of all players and the ball. With this data it could count the number of players of the defensive team which are behind the ball to determine the *Fall Back*. As the pressing index, this number could be emitted periodically.

Figure 4 illustrates the workflow formed by deploying the *Kickoff Detection Worker*, the *Area Detection Worker*, the *Ball Possession Worker*, the *Defensive Play Phase Worker*, the *Pressing Analysis Worker*, and the *Fall Back Worker*.

Table 4. Schema of and example for ball possession change event stream

Schema	ts;playerId;teamId;matchId;playerX;playerY;playerZ;ballX; ballY;ballZ; numPlayersNearerToGoal;type
Example	3822031;A5;A;413237;-31.521;26.916;0.0;-32.454;27.508;0.0;5;vel

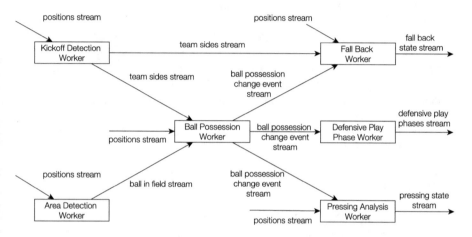

Fig. 4. Workflow for implementing the *Defensive Play* stack in STREAMTEAM

3   Discussion

Football is ever evolving. Our concepts and the preliminary performance model that resulted from Sects. 2.1 and 2.2 represent the elements that the six coaches we have interviewed more or less take into consideration when taking tactical decisions before a match. We assume that these are rather general concepts in football and we plan to further explore this in our future work.

In football, there are many other contexts in which decisions have to be taken, e.g., player and talent development, or training management. Our approach could also be used to extend to other areas of decision-making in football.

The limitation of the analysis system we propose is given by the capacity to detect concepts in the underlying sensor stream. If only positional data of players are available, it is not possible to implement a continuous state like for instance *Orientation* due to a lack of information on the players direction of view and the orientation of the body. Moreover, without information on the referees' decisions (e.g., via a referee stream) match interruptions are difficult to detect.

4 Conclusions

The main goal of this paper is to show a way to close the gap between mental concepts used by the coach in decision-making processes in football and the objective data that is provided by commercial data services or the sport science community. We presented a systematic approach to extract football-specific concepts and to consistently implement them in a customized information system.

With such a match analysis system coaches and analysts are able to answer specific questions using their own concepts as these are represented in the data.

The transfer to other sports is one of the major advantages of the presented approach. As STREAMTEAM is built-up in a very generic way, there is no significant effort needed to create a new version of STREAMTEAM for another sport.

Moreover, the atomic events, phases, and continuous states should be retrievable in an intuitive manner. For this purpose, we have proposed SPORTSENSE [9], a component that lets users intuitively query for video scenes which show events, event cascades, and ball or player motion paths by means of drawing sketches. In our future work, we plan to extend SPORTSENSE with new query types to support answering all the questions we have gathered from the interviews.

Acknowledgements. This work has been partly supported by the Hasler Foundation in the context of the project STREAMTEAM, contract no. 16074.

References

1. Andrienko, G., Andrienko, N., Budziak, G., Dykes, J., Fuchs, G., von Landesberger, T., Weber, H.: Visual analysis of pressure in football. Data Min. Knowl. Discov. **31**(6), 1793–1839 (2017). https://doi.org/10.1007/s10618-017-0513-2

2. Drust, B., Green, M.: Science and football: evaluating the influence of science on performance. J. Sport. Sci. **31**(13), 1377–1382 (2013). https://doi.org/10.1080/02640414.2013.828544

3. Duch, J., Waitzman, J.S., Amaral, L.A.N.: Quantifying the performance of individual players in a team activity. PLoS ONE **5**(6), e10,937 (2010). https://doi.org/10.1371/journal.pone.0010937

4. Fernandez, J., Bornn, L.: Wide open spaces: a statistical technique for measuring space creation in professional soccer. In: MIT Sloan Sports Analytics Conference (2018)

5. Kuckartz, U.: Qualitative Inhaltsanalyse. Methoden, Praxis, Computerunterstützung, 4 edn. Beltz Verlagsgruppe, Weinheim (2018)

6. Link, D., Hoernig, M.: Individual ball possession in soccer. PLoS ONE **12**(7), e0179,953 (2017). https://doi.org/10.1371/journal.pone.0179953

7. Mackenzie, R., Cushion, C.: Performance analysis in football: a critical review and implications for future research. J. Sport. Sci. **31**(6), 639–676 (2013). https://doi.org/10.1080/02640414.2012.746720

8. Noghabi, S.A., Paramasivam, K., Pan, Y., Ramesh, N., Bringhurst, J., Gupta, I., Campbell, R.H.: Samza: stateful scalable stream processing at LinkedIn. Proc. VLDB Endow. **10**(12), 1634–1645 (2017). https://doi.org/10.14778/3137765.3137770

9. Probst, L., Al Kabary, I., Lobo, R., Rauschenbach, F., Schuldt, H., Seidenschwarz, P., Rumo, M.: SportSense: user interface for sketch-based spatio-temporal team sports video scene retrieval. In: Proceedings of the 1st Workshop on User Interface for Spatial and Temporal Data Analysis, Tokyo, Japan. CEUR-WS (2018)
10. Probst, L., Brix, F., Schuldt, H., Rumo, M.: Real-time football analysis with StreamTeam. In: Proceedings of the 11th ACM International Conference on Distributed and Event-based Systems, Barcelona, Spain, pp. 319–322. ACM (2017). https://doi.org/10.1145/3093742.3095089
11. Probst, L., Rauschenbach, F., Schuldt, H., Seidenschwarz, P., Rumo, M.: Integrated real-time data stream analysis and sketch-based video retrieval in team sports. In: Proceedings of the 2018 IEEE International Conference on Big Data, pp. 548–555. IEEE (2018). https://doi.org/10.1109/BigData.2018.8622592
12. Spearman, W.: Beyond expected goals. In: MIT Sloan Sports Analytics Conference (2018)

Evaluating the Contribution of Foreign Players by Player Contribution Indicator in Football Leagues

Junxian Jiang and Hui Zhang[✉]

Department of Sport Science, College of Education,
Zhejiang University, Hangzhou, China
{junxian_jiang, zhang_hui}@zju.edu.cn

Abstract. This paper aims to develop and validate the Player Contribution Indicator (PCI) based on players' playing time per game and the point earned per game. At the same time, using the PCI to measure the foreign players' contribution during a season and to roughly evaluate the comprehensive contribution of foreign players. And the main league studied is Premier League and LaLiga, two of the Europe's Top 5 Leagues. Through analyzing the comparison among the PCI of foreign players and ranking the contribution level of each countries, it is shown that the general situation of foreign players in the league. And it has practical useful for the following research on player contribution level, foreign players' policy setting and league level comparison.

Keywords: Football · Player Contribution Indicator · Foreign players

1 Introduction

1.1 Background

At present, Europe's Top 5 Leagues all have foreign players, and are being joined by an increasing number of players from other parts of the world after the release of the "Bosman-ruling". Most researchers evaluate players' contribution in one specific league, while there is little comparison among different leagues (Dellal 2010). Some researches compare the contribution of individual players using technical and tactical indices (Alexandre 2010).

1.2 Object

The main reach object of this page are foreign player. Normally speaking, the players called as foreigners are not born in the host country of the league. Therefore, this paper defines foreign players as players born in countries outside the host country of the league in which they are playing, and uses their country of birth as the only indicator of nationality statistics. This definition also applies to dual nationality players. It's worth noting that, this definition is not valid for players who have represented the official adult national team in the international game. The players represent their official

© Springer Nature Switzerland AG 2020
M. Lames et al. (Eds.): IACSS 2019, AISC 1028, pp. 28–35, 2020.
https://doi.org/10.1007/978-3-030-35048-2_4

national team to attend international games whose country will be regarded as the only indicator of their nationality statistics.

For example, Diego Costa, currently playing for the Atletico Madrid Athletic Club in La Liga as a centre-forward, was born in Brazil and has double-level nationality in Brazil and Spain. However, since he has represented the Spanish official national team, he will not be regarded as a foreign player in this article, but a native Spanish player.

All foreign players in squad are recorded including the Winter transfer and the Summer transfer, even if the player never show up in the match during the season. But the player never used in the season don't make sense to PCI.

1.3   Aim

How to evaluate the comprehensive contribution of foreign players in different leagues has raised debate in football. People are eager to know which country's oversea player are the best. On this basis, researchers can have a deeper understanding of the relationship between oversea players and resident players. And it also make contribution to measure policies about the restriction of foreign players.

However, it is difficult to evaluate the comprehensive contribution of players with some simple indices. At the present stage, most of the evaluation systems are not perfect. People tend to adopt different evaluation indexes for players in different positions in the same system, so that the score of forward players is often greater than that of goalkeeper. It's not easy to find a metric that works for all players. Therefore, this passage put forward PCI composed by simple calculation to solve this problem.

The rest of this passage is organized as follows. Section 2 describes the data and method. Section 3 conclude the main result. At the last, the Sect. 4 provide the overall conclusion of the passage and discuss some phenomenon.

2   Method and Data

2.1   Method

The PCI (Player contribution Indicator) is composed of two parts: the ratio of contribution (R) and the points earned per game (P). The formula is as follows:

$$PCI = \sum_{i=1}^{n} (R_i * P_i) \tag{1}$$

n is the total number of the match during the season and i refers to the number i match $(i = 1, 2, 3, \ldots, n)$.

The Ratio of Contribution (R)
This index is based on players' playing time. Based on the assumption that the players' appearance times are strongly related to their contribution without regard to injuries or midseason transfers. As we know, in modern football, teams have three substitutions per game, excluding extra time match. At least eight players of the starting line-up in each game need to play 90 min. The substitution of player mainly depends on the player's contribution on the field, including tactical needs, physical level, mental state,

skill level. At the same time, "Football is round, anything is possible", the football game is a dynamic process that the state of the match changes rapidly. Once a player is on the field, even for a minute, he becomes part of the game. Only when the player is on the field can he show his value. He could be a key player in the game, he could be the sinner of the game, but that's only going to happen if he gets a chance to play. In other words, the higher the quality the player shows, the more appearance time the player got.

Theoretically speaking, each player has the same total appearances time over the whole season—if the player does not miss a game and plays the whole game (a notional 90 min per game). The more playing time a player has, the more chances the player has to perform. As a result, the players' appearances time could be used as the index to evaluate players' contribution and is not affected by the players' position.

Under current football rules, each side has 11 players on the pitch. No matter how the players are substituted, each side is limited to 11 players. Even if a player is shown the red card, he still has a place of these 11 players. What's more, the legal time of a match is 90 min in total. Game injure-time is also essentially set to keep the game close to 90 min. So the total time for each team per game is 990 min (90 min * 11).

The ratio of contribution is equal to the playing time per game divided by 990 min. The formula is as follows:

$$R = \frac{playingtime}{90 * 11} \tag{2}$$

The Points Earned Per Game (P)

Previously, it was very difficult to evaluate players' contribution by the same index because different positions have different kinds of data. Generally speaking, the defenders have more data on the defensive side, such as clearance and interception and the strikers have more data on the offensive side, such as goal and shoot. Save or pass, which contributes more to the team? It's hard to say.

Football is a team sport, instead of an individual sport. The modern football stresses the integrity, the first-class football team must have both attack and defense, and the whole team members participate in all links. That is to say, even if the team position is clear, the goalkeeper will also participate in the assist, the striker will also participate in the clearance. As long as the players are on the field, their every minute and every move is likely to contribute to the team. So how can these contributions be measured?

For football match, goals are at the heart of the game. All the players want the team to score as many goals as possible and concede as few as possible. But in the end, there is only one measure of a team's ultimate success, and that is the outcome of the game. A score of 1–0 is always better than a score of 5–5. Because the team gets a win instead of a draw. A score of 0–0 is always better than a score of 0–1. Because the team gets a draw instead of a failure.

Most modern football leagues use the point system, win 3 points, draw 1 point and lose 0 points. The teams are ranked by the league table at the end of all games of the season. Points are used as the criterion to measure the success of a team. Teams that want to be at the top of the table must get more points. The players, as part of the team, make their contribution to the team to get more point. Therefore, Points earned per game can be used to evaluate a player's contribution. At the same time, this indicator is relatively easy to obtain, and apply to all positions of the players.

2.2   Data Collection

This study collected the data of all foreign players' appearance time and League table per round in Premier League within the period of 2013/2014-2017/2018. All the data was collected from the website of Transfermarkt (https://www.transfermarkt.com/).

3   Result

3.1   LaLiga

LaLiga is contested by 20 teams during the season. The basic situation about foreign players and PCI of the LaLiga between the season 2013/2014 to the season 2017/2018 is as follows (Table 1).

LaLiga has the fewest foreign players among the Europe's Top 5 Leagues. The number of foreign player and PCI generally fluctuates widely.

Table 1. Basic situation and PCI of LaLiga

League	Season	Countries	Foreigners	Total PCI
LaLiga	2013/2014	56	236	420.6455
LaLiga	2014/2015	55	215	470.1667
LaLiga	2015/2016	60	238	466.9455
LaLiga	2016/2017	50	250	476.5111
LaLiga	2017/2018	54	253	459.2485
Average		55	238.4	458.7034

The PCI ranking top 35 of foreign player in LaLiga is as follows (Fig. 1):

The number one country is Argentina with more than 30 players in each season, including soccer superstar Lionel Messi. Brazil, France and Portugal came in second, third and fourth. These countries have a lot of foreign players in LaLiga. The PCI of the top five countries is at a very high level and there is a big gap between them. From the sixth place, the gap between the former and the latter begin to narrow.

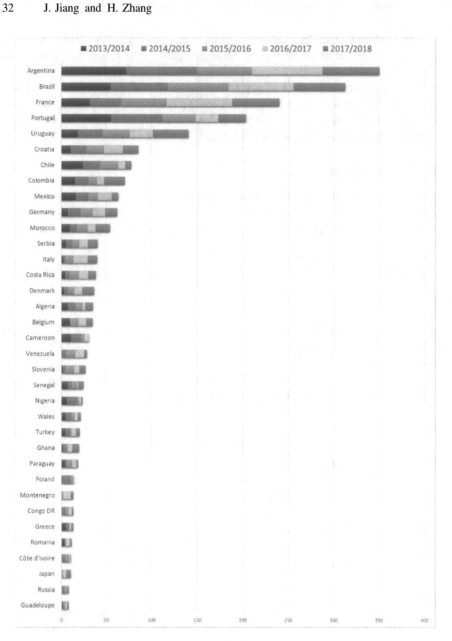

Fig. 1. PCI of foreign players in LaLiga during 2013/2014–2017/2018 (Top35)

Surprisingly, the continent with the most seats in the top 10 is not Europe, but South America with half of them. Overall, Latin American players make the most contribution to LaLiga, followed by European players and African players. In Asia, only Japan ranked in the top 35, with a relatively low contribution.

3.2   Premier League

The Premier League (EPL) is contested by 20 clubs during the season. The basic situation about foreign players and PCI of the Premier League between the season 2013/2014 to the season 2017/2018 is as follows (Table 2).

Thanks to the loose foreign players' policy, the Premier League has the largest number of foreign players in the Europe's Top 5 Leagues. So the level of PCI is much higher than other leagues. The PCI of Premier League has fluctuated greatly in recent years.

Table 2. Basic situation and PCI of Premier League

League	Season	Countries	Foreigners	Total PCI
Premier League	2013/2014	71	420	737.2162
Premier League	2014/2015	65	390	702.4293
Premier League	2015/2016	68	413	729.3455
Premier League	2016/2017	62	379	724.6475
Premier League	2017/2018	67	381	713.7455
Average		66.6	396.6	721.4768

The PCI ranking top 50 of foreign player in Premier League is as follows (Fig. 2):

The situation in the premier league is markedly different from that in LaLiga. Most of the top 10 countries are in Europe, with Spain, France and Belgium in the top three. Brazil and Argentina are the only South American countries in the top 10, ranking fourth and fifth. Notably, Brazil's PCI is only about half as high as Spain's. The top three, Spain, France and Belgium, account for a large part of the overall PCI of foreign players in the premier league.

Overall, most of the premier league's foreign player comes from European Union nations. This is probably due to the convenience of EU visas to play in Premier League.

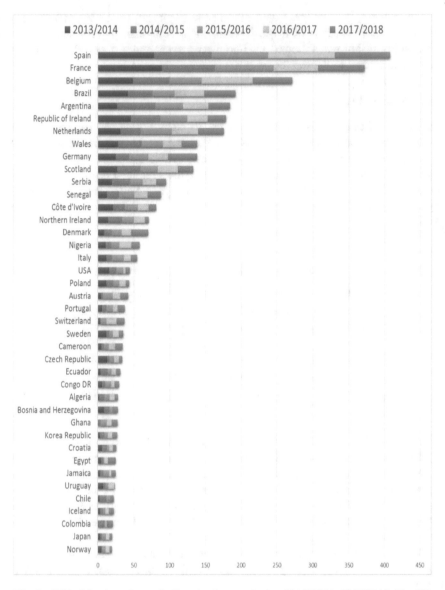

Fig. 2. PCI of foreign players in Premier League during 2013/2014–2017/2018 (Top50)

4 Conclusion and Discussion

The passage evaluates the contribution of foreign players in different leagues with simple indices by building PCI model.

Through PCI, we can have a deeper understanding of the foreign players' situation in each league. On this basis, this will help people to carry out more research about foreign players.

From the national level, which country's players make more contribution in the Premier League and LaLiga? To answer this question, the Leagues' PCI were split into each country and add up by season. Surprisingly, the result is very stable during the 5 seasons. The top 5 of the Premier League and LaLiga are European countries and southern America. In particular, the PCI of European countries in the premier league is much larger than that of other continents. That means that the migration of football workforce in Europe's Top-level Leagues is increasingly concentrated in European countries and parts of South America, with less talent from other continents. Does this phenomenon play a role in the development of football in Europe and other continents? What kind of effect they are? In recent years the World Cup finals have been dominated by European teams and most of the player were come from the Europe's Top 5 Leagues. The 2018 World Cup winner, France, is the team with the highest CPI combined in LaLiga and the premier league. Whether there is a certain relationship between PCI and national team strength? This is a direction worthy of our consideration and future research.

This passage is the building of PCI to evaluate the contribution of foreign players. With the PCI, we can easily calculate a player's contribution in a season. It can also be used to compare the differences between different players, different teams and foreign player from different countries. Perhaps the greatest contribution of PCI is to give a fresh perspective on the players' contributions to the game. In the following research, it is hoped that PCI can be used as a sub-index to evaluate players' level and game performance.

References

1. Sargent, J., Bedford, A.: Evaluating australian football league player contributions using interactive network simulation. J. Sport. Sci. Med. **12**(1), 116 (2013)
2. Dellal, A., Chamari, K., et al.: Comparison of physical and technical performance in European soccer match-play: FA Premier League and La Liga. Eur. J. Sport. Sci. **11**(1), 51–59 (2011)
3. Suzuki, K., Ohmori, K.: Effectiveness of FIFA/Coca-Cola world ranking in predicting the results of FIFA world CupTM finals. Footb. Sci. **5**, 18–25 (2008)
4. Cafagna, V., Donati, F.: Impact on competitive balance from allowing foreign players in a sports league: evidence from European soccer. Kyklos **63**(4), 546–557 (2010)
5. Frick, B.: Globalization and factor mobility: the impact of the "Bosman-Ruling" on player migration in professional soccer. J. Sport. Econ. **10**(1), 88–106 (2009)
6. Adcroft, A., Madichie, N.: Management implications of foreign players in the English Premiership League football. Manag. Decis. **47**(1), 24–50 (2009)

Performance of Performance Indicators in Football

Tiago Russomanno[1]([✉]) [iD], Daniel Linke[2] [iD], Max Geromiller[2],
and Martin Lames[2] [iD]

[1] University of Brasilia, Campus Universitário Darcy Ribeiro, Brasília, Brazil
tiagorussomanno@unb.br
[2] TU München, Georg-Brauchle-Ring 62, 80809 Munich, Germany

Abstract. Performance indicators (PIs) play a key role in today's sports analytics. In this paper we examine the performance of performance indicators with respect to (match)day-to-day stability and predictive validity for final ranking. A sample of 279 football matches of the German Bundesliga in the Season 2016/2017 was analyzed. Inter-day correlations were computed per PI using Pearson correlations. The distribution of 450 inter-day correlations per PI was analyzed. Spearman's rank correlations between season mean values of the PIs and final ranking were calculated as validity check. Also, the Pearson intercorrelations between the PIs were analyzed for exploring their mutual relationships. The results show rather low correlations with the highest median correlation of 0.43 for number of completed passes. The highest predictive values (0.794–0.771) were found for traditional PIs like number of passes as well as for more recently introduced Packing PIs. Inter-correlations reveal that the more recent PIs are very highly correlated with traditional ones. The findings support the view of matches as not repeatable, dynamic interaction processes with emergent behavior rather than being predictable by summative PIs.

Keywords: Performance analysis · Modeling · Football · Performance indicators

1 Introduction

Performance indicators (PIs) play a key role in today's sports analytics, traditionally in US-sports but increasingly also in other game sports like football [1]. In training and coaching, PIs play an important role mostly as starting point for a more in-depth qualitative game analysis [2]. A variety of indicators was created to explain behavior and performance in football. Only recently, with the advent of positional data in football, totally new families of PIs came into reach.

A closer look at PIs in football reveals a development towards an increasing complexity. Whereas in earlier days simple counts and percentages in the action domain and aggregations of kinematic variables in the position domain were prevalent, today's research focuses on performance indicators that try to operationalize complex constructs used by practitioners to analyze football with, e.g. [3].

© Springer Nature Switzerland AG 2020
M. Lames et al. (Eds.): IACSS 2019, AISC 1028, pp. 36–44, 2020.
https://doi.org/10.1007/978-3-030-35048-2_5

There are two basic interpretations of performance indicators [4]: On the one side they may be seen as pure descriptions of what was happening on the pitch, on the other side they may be taken as indicators of stable properties of strengths and weaknesses of teams and players. The first view poses almost no methodological problems: If the measurements show a sufficient accuracy (observer agreement for event-based PIs; physical accuracy for kinematic ones) we have valid descriptions for behavior taking place in the pitch. This attitude is frequently, sometimes unconsciously, extended towards taking PIs as indicators for stable properties like tactical, technical or athletic performance levels or strengths and weaknesses of the athletes [4].

We find this quite widespread, for example in sports media when PIs are used to identify the "better" team. In sports practice though, one has to adopt this notion when the intention is to derive hints for training from match performance (a frequent aim of practical performance analysis). In this case, one looks for properties of the players that explain match behavior and makes these targets of training if room for improvement is expected. This notion is much more demanding from an assessment point of view, though. If PIs are seen as indicators of stable properties of the athletes one must postulate a certain stability, which is an aspect of reliability, and above all a relevance for success, which is an aspect of validity [4].

This discussion touches the question of appropriate models for football matches. Do we see them as unique dynamic interaction processes with emerging behavior patterns, or as being determined by the two sets of performance prerequisites of the opponents? In the first case PIs would be just descriptions of behavior, in the latter they are indicators for stable properties of the players.

There are only few studies that focus on a comparison of performance indicators for example with respect to their capability of predicting success in matches or over a season, e.g. [5]. They mostly correlate the final outcome of a tournament or a season with the PIs and only occasionally inter-correlations between PIs are studied.

This study aims at analyzing a set of performance indicators representative of traditional and recent ones. Two aspects are studied. First, the question of stability is addressed in analyzing inter-match day correlations of each PI over a season in professional football. Second, the predictive validity of the PIs is scrutinized by correlating the season means of the PIs with the final ranking of the teams.

2 Methods

2.1 Sample

A sample of 279 football matches of the German Bundesliga in the Season 2016/2017 was analyzed. This is the full season with some matches missing because of non-reported PIs, which were list-wise excluded. The sample consists of the 31 match days with complete data. Overall, 8,928 PIs were collected.

2.2   Performance Indicators

The following PIs were sampled (source, if no other is given: www.opta.de):

- Goals scored (Goals): Reference indicator for maximum success of a team
- Expected goals (Expec. Goals): Sum of number of shots in certain situation classes multiplied with scoring probability of that class, gives an expected value for the number of goals scored (www.alexrathke.net).
- Shots: Number of shots directed at goal
- Shots on goal: Number of shots hitting goal
- Packing: Sum of opponent players overcome by each successful pass
- Packing defence (Pack. Def.): Sum of players in opponent's defence overcome by each successful pass
- Passes: Number of passes
- Passes completed (Passes Com.): Number of completed passes
- Rank: Final ranking of team
- Rank per day: Ranking of team at match day

These PIs were recorded as summative statistics per match and per team thus resulting per PI in two variables, one for the team under consideration and one for the respective opponent, e.g. "passes" and "passes opp.".

2.3   Statistical Procedures

Statistical analyses include descriptive statistics (mean, standard deviation, max, min, coefficient of variation (CV)) for all PIs. Inter-day Spearman correlations are calculated for each PI ($n = 18$ teams); 31 match days yield 450 inter-day correlations. The distributions per PI of the inter-day correlations were described with percentiles (median, 25%-Quartile, 75%-Quartile, max, min, interquartile range (IR)) because of scale properties of correlations. To analyze criterion or predictive validity, Spearman's rank correlations between the season's mean of the PIs and the final ranking of the teams were calculated. Moreover, the inter-correlations between the PIs were calculated using Pearson's correlation.

Since all data were retrieved from publicly available sources, no ethics statement is required.

3   Results

3.1   Descriptive Statistics of PIs

Table 1 shows the descriptive statistics of the PIs under scrutiny. For each of the 18 teams the statistics for the season means of the PIs are depicted.

As we have for each match the value for a PI and the PI of the opponent (PI opp.), the overall means per team for PI and PI opp. are in principle equal. The small differences in Table 1 are due to missing values that may affect PI and PI opp. slightly differently. This does not hold for the other statistics as we have team specific effects on PI and PI opp.

The CVs range from 7.75% to 33.94% with only two of the PIs showing a CV below 10% that is seen in economics as a threshold for a stable measurement [6]. In performance analysis, sometimes even a threshold below 5% is demanded for a stable variable [7]. The highest CV is found for goals scored followed by the number of completed passes. The highest stability is found in the packing statistics of the opponents.

Table 1. Descriptive statistics of season mean for each team (n = 18) per PI. Note that PI and PI Opp. must have the same mean except for small differences due to missing values.

PI	Mean	StDev	Min	Max	CV
Goals	1.44	0.49	0.88	2.69	33.94
Goals Opp.	1.45	0.33	0.66	1.97	23.16
Expec. Goals	1.26	0.28	0.92	1.96	22.42
Expec. Goals Opp.	1.26	0.22	0.86	1.72	17.40
Shots	12.39	2.07	9.94	18.03	16.69
Shots Opp.	12.39	1.96	8.88	16.09	15.80
Shots on Goal	4.39	0.96	2.94	6.66	21.79
Shots on Goal Opp.	4.39	0.85	2.66	5.81	19.27
Passes	447.15	95.41	310.84	710.56	21.34
Passes Opp.	447.14	56.10	315.63	533.22	12.55
Passes Com.	343.00	99.84	211.91	620.34	29.10
Passes Com. Opp.	343.10	54.87	228.41	430.41	15.99
Packing	283.87	46.94	218.97	418.13	16.54
Packing Opp.	283.86	23.74	233.00	329.97	8.36
Packing Def.	38.94	5.32	30.32	49.23	13.66
Packing Def. Opp.	38.94	3.02	34.48	47.00	7.75

3.2   Inter-day Correlations

In Table 2 the distributions of the 450 inter-day correlations are given with percentiles.

Table 2. Descriptive statistics for the inter-day Spearman correlations for each PI (n = 18 teams; 450 correlations per PI).

PI	Median	25%	75%	Min	Max	IR
Rank per day	0.88	0.80	0.95	−0.37	0.99	0.15
Goals	0.08	−0.08	0.25	−0.55	0.72	0.33
Goals Opp.	0.03	−0.14	0.23	−0.71	0.75	0.37
Expec. Goals	0.11	−0.05	0.28	−0.64	0.76	0.33
Expec. Goals Opp.	0.10	−0.07	0.26	−0.50	0.72	0.33
Shots	0.15	−0.03	0.29	−0.48	0.76	0.32
Shots Opp.	0.11	−0.02	0.26	−0.63	0.84	0.28
Shots on Goal	0.11	−0.05	0.28	−0.66	0.76	0.33

(*continued*)

Table 2. (*continued*)

PI	Median	25%	75%	Min	Max	IR
Shots on Goal Opp.	0.12	−0.05	0.25	−0.58	0.78	0.33
Passes	0.40	0.28	0.52	−0.04	0.82	0.24
Passes Opp.	0.15	0.00	0.33	−0.43	0.75	0.32
Passes Com.	0.43	0.32	0.55	0.03	0.86	0.23
Passes Com. Opp.	0.12	−0.03	0.31	−0.52	0.75	0.34
Packing	0.39	0.27	0.54	−0.19	0.81	0.26
Packing Opp.	0.09	−0.07	0.28	−0.63	0.71	0.35
Pack. Def.	0.13	−0.04	0.28	−0.69	0.68	0.32
Pack. Def. Opp.	0.02	−0.15	0.19	−0.70	0.69	0.33

Day-to-day variability of PIs must be described as high. The median inter-day correlations exceed .70, the common threshold for a retest-reliability [8], only in the case of rank by day (.88) indicating that the place in the table becomes rather stable in the course of a season. Behind this, the highest medians for the inter-day correlations are found for completed passes (.43), passes (.40) and packing (.39). Only the medians of the correlations for rank by day and completed passes are significantly different from zero (n = 18).

3.3   Correlations with Final Ranking

Figure 1 shows the Spearman correlation between the means of the PIs and the final ranking at the end of the season. The absolute values of the correlations are given. PIs are sorted according to descending correlation for the team's PIs.

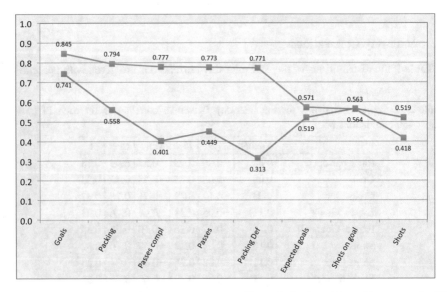

Fig. 1. Spearman's correlations between mean PIs and final ranking (blue = team's PI; orange = opponent's PI).

The highest predictive value for a team's final ranking is found for the goals scored by the team (.845). Behind this, there are four PIs within a very small range between .794 and .771: Packing, Passes completed, Passes and Packing defence. There is a considerable gap to Expected goals and Shots on goal, the lowest predictive value is found for the number of shots. The opponent's PIs are found in the interval between .563 and .313, except for the opponent's number of goals with .741.

3.4 Inter-correlations Between PIs

In Table 3 the Spearman inter-correlations between the season's means of the PIs of the 18 teams are given. In general, we have medium to high inter-correlations; only few of them fail to be significant.

Correlations between a team's PI and the corresponding PI of the opponent are negatively correlated, for example shots with shots of opponent (−.750). Moreover, taken absolute values a team's PI is stronger correlated with any other PI than with the corresponding PI of the opponent, for example shots with shots on goal (.871), but shots with opponent's shots on goal (−.505).

Table 3. Spearman inter-correlations between season's mean PIs for the 18 teams (p < .05 if |r| > .40; p < .01 if |r| > .54)

	Goals	Goals Opp.	Expec. goals	Expec. goals Opp.	Shots	Shots Opp.	Shots on Goal	Shots on Goal Opp.	Passes	Passes Opp.	Passes Com.	Passes com. Opp.	Packing	Packing Opp.	Pack. Def.	Pack. Def. Opp.
Goals		-,601	,739	-,605	,617	-,590	,807	-,366	,783	-,584	,770	-,537	,816	-,605	,828	-,311
Goals Opp.	-,601		-,626	,805	-,509	,736	-,390	,749	-,608	,561	-,640	,499	-,588	,701	-,583	,522
Expec. goals	,739	-,626		-,789	,891	-,833	,808	-,598	,781	-,917	,787	-,856	,796	-,754	,775	-,265
Expec. goals Opp.	-,605	,805	-,789		-,738	,903	-,631	,749	-,701	,787	-,699	,728	-,610	,882	-,503	,519
Shots	,617	-,509	,891	-,738		-,750	,871	-,505	,659	-,860	,659	-,825	,657	-,736	,666	-,263
Shots Opp.	-,590	,736	-,833	,903	-,750		-,669	,773	-,697	,872	-,709	,872	-,591	,818	-,538	,379
Shots on Goal	,807	-,390	,808	-,631	,871	-,669		-,359	,721	-,760	,694	-,762	,722	-,708	,737	-,294
Shots on Goal Opp.	-,366	,749	-,598	,749	-,505	,773	-,359		-,524	,681	-,533	,687	-,432	,765	-,364	,374
Passes	,783	-,608	,781	-,701	,659	-,697	,721	-,524		-,721	,992	-,612	,940	-,688	,730	-,199
Passes Opp.	-,584	,561	-,917	,787	-,860	,872	-,760	,681	-,721		-,728	,959	-,655	,845	-,556	,321
Passes Com.	,770	-,640	,787	-,699	,659	-,709	,694	-,533	,992	-,728		-,610	,934	-,688	,723	-,209
Passes com. Opp.	-,537	,499	-,856	,728	-,825	,872	-,762	,687	-,612	,959	-,610		-,554	,785	-,552	,327
Packing	,816	-,588	,796	-,610	,657	-,591	,722	-,432	,940	-,655	,934	-,554		-,571	,872	-,108
Packing Opp.	-,605	,701	-,754	,882	-,736	,818	-,708	,765	-,688	,845	-,688	,785	-,571		-,426	,637
Pack. Def.	,828	-,583	,775	-,503	,666	-,538	,737	-,364	,730	-,556	,723	-,552	,872	-,426		-,135
Pack. Def. Opp.	-,311	,522	-,265	,519	-,263	,379	-,294	,374	-,199	,321	-,209	,327	-,108	,637	-,135	

The mean number of goals scored per match correlates highest with the own packing PIs (Packing defence: .828; Packing: .816). Interestingly this is (a bit) higher than shots on goal (.807) and expected goals (.739).

Expected goals were only recently introduced as PI probably because shooting positions are required for their calculation. This indicator is highly correlated with the number of shots (.891) and, interestingly, by the opponent's number of passes (−.917) and completed passes (−.856).

Packing is a rather recent performance indicator as well. Here we have strikingly high correlations with number of passes (.940) and completed passes (.934).

4 Discussion

In sports analytics, we find a wealth of PIs with new ones continuously suggested in literature. Thus, it is important to check the performance of new and existing PIs in the sense of their reliability and validity. In this study, a sample of traditional (shots, shots on goal, passes, and passes completed) as well as recent PIs (expected goals, packing, packing defence) was collected for a whole season of German Bundesliga except 3 match days with non-reported PIs. The aspect of inter-day stability was checked for reliability, and criterion referenced validity was checked by correlating the season's means of the 18 teams per PI with the number of goals scored and the final ranking. The internal structure of all PIs was assessed with their inter-correlation matrix.

Descriptive results show a high variation of the PIs between the teams indicated by 87.5% of the coefficients of variation above 10%, which is a threshold acknowledged for stable variables [6, 7]. This means that the teams of German Bundesliga differ largely with respect to their average PIs over a season, which is a well-desired property as PIs should explain differences between teams.

Results for inter-day correlations of the PIs show a high intra-seasonal variation of all PIs. Except for the day-to-day ranking with a median correlation of .880 all PIs fail to reach the minimum threshold of reproducibility of .70 for assessing a stable property [8]. In only three cases (passes, completed passes, packing) the median correlation indicates at least a weak effect size > .20 according to Cohen [9]. These were exactly the variables with the highest absolute frequencies. For these three PIs the interquartile interval accounts for between 53.4 and 66.7% median, which indicates a high dispersion in the distribution. For the other PIs this percentage is much higher, at least 200%. Taken together, results on the inter-day correlations show that there is high fluctuation from match day to match day. The level of a performance indicator on one match day is at best only weakly connected with its level on any other day.

Controlling for criterion referenced validity by correlating the mean values of the PIs for a season with the final ranking of the teams resulted in a quite high (.845) but rather trivial correlation for the average number of goals scored per match. It is interesting to note that more recently developed PIs perform only as good as (packing: .794) or even worse (Expected goals: .571) than traditional PIs. The PIs with the best predictive power account for between 59 and 63% of the variance in final ranking. This shows on one hand that these PIs account for a massive part of the overall performance, on the other hand it is obvious that they are far away from explaining overall performance perfectly. This holds interestingly also for the average number of goals scored per match (71% common variance with final ranking).

The most interesting finding from the study of inter-correlations between PIs is that the recently introduced PIs that make some (in the case of packing) use of positional data are very highly correlated to traditional PIs, e.g. packing with number of passes (.940) and expected goals with number of shots (.891). In general, we find quite high inter-correlations between the different PIs. An explorative factor analysis with a general factor model demonstrated that three quarters of the PIs had a commonality of over 80%, i.e. they were explained to a large extend by a general factor. A general factor comes up for 75% of the total variance, indicating that all the different PIs examined assess to a great extent the same construct.

There are some limitations of this study, however. It would of course be of great value if one had a full sample of PIs for a season without missing match days. Then, the sample of performance indicators represents only a small fraction of indicators on the market comprehending not at all indicators of physical performance like distance covered, high intensive running and others. Also, it would be interesting to compare betting odds to PIs as recently suggested in [10]. A larger sample of matches than the 279 in our sample would be desirable, also. Maybe the situation changes from year to year or in different leagues.

5 Conclusions

The examination of the performance of performance indicators in football shows that neither there is a sufficient stability of these measurements between the days of a season nor an impressive predictive capability for the final (and for the clubs decisive) ranking in the league. Moreover, there is a large overlap between the constructs each PI under scrutiny is representing, as shown by the efficacy of a general factor model. It is by no way justified to assume that new PIs add much value to the existing traditional ones.

The results speak very much in favour of a purely descriptive function of PIs being valid only as assessments of behaviour that took place in the pitch each match. Lacking match-to-match stability and only moderate predictive validity for the final ranking of the teams underline this interpretation.

What the notion of football and game sports in general is concerned, the results give a clear argument for perceiving game sports as unique, dynamic interaction processes with uncontrollable chance impact [11] rather than the output of a comparison between two sets of performance prerequisites seen as stable properties of teams and athletes. So, at the time being, conclusions on stable strengths and weaknesses of teams and players have to rely on qualitative analyses [2] rather than proficient PIs. It will be interesting to see whether future PIs will be able to overcome these problems.

References

1. Sampaio, J., Leite, N.: Performance indicators in game sports. In: McGarry, T., O'Donoghue, P., Sampaio, J. (eds.) Routledge Handbook of Sports Performance Analysis, pp. 115–126. Routledge, London (2013)
2. Lames, M., Hansen, G.: Designing observational systems to support top-level teams in game sports. Int. J. Perform. Anal. 1(1), 85–91 (2001)
3. Link, D., Lang, S., Seidenschwarz, P.: Real time quantification of dangerousity in football using spatiotemporal tracking data. PLoS ONE 11(12), e0168768 (2016). https://doi.org/10.1371/journal.pone.0168768
4. Lames, M., McGarry, T.: On the search for reliable performance indicators in game sports. Int. J. Perform. Anal. Sport 7(1), 62–79 (2007)

5. Harrop, K., Nevill, A.: Performance indicators that predict success in an English professional League One soccer team. Int. J. Perform. Anal. Sport **14**(3), 907–920 (2014)
6. Statistisches Bundesamt: Intrahandelsstatistik. Wirtsch. Stat. **59**(9), 784–789 (2008)
7. Buchheit, M., Lefebvre, B., Laursen, P.B., Ahmaidi, S.: Reliability, usefulness, and validity of the 30–15 intermittent ice test in young elite ice hockey players. J. Strength Cond. Res. **25**, 1457–1464 (2011)
8. Lienert, G.A.: Testaufbau und Testanalyse. Beltz, Weinheim (1969)
9. Cohen, J.: Statistical Power Analysis for the Behavioral Sciences, 2nd edn. Erlbaum, Hillsdale (1988)
10. Wunderlich, F., Memmert, D.: Analysis of the predictive qualities of betting odds and FIFA World Ranking: evidence from the 2006, 2010 and 2014 Football World Cups. J. Sport Sci. **34**(24), 2176–2184 (2016)
11. Lames, M.: Chance involvement in goal scoring in football – an empirical approach. Ger. J. Exerc. Sport Res. **48**(2), 278–286 (2018)

A Multi-dimensional Analytical System of Table Tennis Matches

Zheng Zhou and Hui Zhang[✉]

Department of Sport Science, College of Education, Zhejiang University,
Hangzhou 310028, Zhejiang, China
{zheng.zhou, zhang_hui}@zju.edu.cn

Abstract. This paper takes 47 technical and tactical indices of 7 categories of table tennis matches, including stroke placements, stroke techniques, stroke positions, game actions, stroke effects, stroke spins and stroke results to construct a multi-dimensional analytical system with data mining algorithm. On this basis, 10 matches between Japanese female player ITO Mima and Chinese players are analyzed systematically. The results show that: (1) The collection system has three main functions, including video monitoring, video editing, technical and tactical information editing; (2) Match data, videos and tactical graphics provided by the analytical system can help players and coaches understand tactics more quickly and meticulously; (3) The effective tactics of ITO Mima are more diverse and aggressive in the receive round; and the main tactic of her is serving the ball to short, and striking with topspin in backhand initiatively (serve round), while in the receive round, attack and topspin in backhand are most obvious technical and tactical features; (4) The application of data mining and modeling in game analysis can reduce the judgment error by human, and make the results more objective and accurate.

Keywords: Table tennis · Multi-dimensional analysis · Elite players

1 Introduction

Table tennis match analysis, which includes descriptive analysis, computer-aided analysis and model analysis, plays an active role in helping coaches and players understand table tennis matches (Fuchs et al. 2018; Zhang et al. 2018). Most of the descriptive analysis adopts the "three-phase evaluation method" in the 1980s which divides each rally into three phases according to the stroke order: the first and third strokes (the phase of serve and attack), the second and fourth strokes (the phase of receive and attack) and the after-the-fourth strokes (the phase of stalemate), and analyzes their scoring rate and usage rate (Wu et al. 1989). Being simple and easy to understand, this method is popular among coaches and players. However, since it doesn't involve the specific techniques and stroke placements of players in the match, it is unable to carry out a deeper diagnosis.

Computer-aided analysis refers to obtaining match statistics and related match videos by manually capturing the characteristics of match indices with computer techniques, which allows coaches and players to get more information about matches

© Springer Nature Switzerland AG 2020
M. Lames et al. (Eds.): IACSS 2019, AISC 1028, pp. 45–52, 2020.
https://doi.org/10.1007/978-3-030-35048-2_6

(Zhang et al. 2010). However, the disadvantage of this method is that it requires a lot of manpower and time, and the video collector needs to have profound professional knowledge of table tennis in order to accurately identify a player's match behavior. Model analysis, such as using neural network and association rules to model and analyze various match indices (Yang and Zhang 2016; Zhang and Zhou 2017), is a popular method in recent years. Its advantage is that this model has higher precision and even has the ability to predict a match, while the disadvantage is that match indices are separated and discussed independently with no connection to each other. Therefore, the collection and analysis of video data (multi-dimensional indices) is still a bottleneck that constrains the development of table tennis match analysis.

In recent years, the Japanese table tennis team has risen quickly. Its men and women players have repeatedly defeated Chinese players, showing striking performances, especially the female Japanese players HIRANO Miu and ITO Mima. HIRANO Miu won the Asian Championships in 2017 after defeating three Chinese players in a row. In 2018, ITO Mima not only defeated Chinese players for many times, but also beat three world champions and Olympic champions of the Chinese team in the Swedish Tour with the same tactics. They have become a main threat to the Chinese team.

This paper attempts to create a table tennis match analysis system to analyze techniques and tactics of ITO Mima in the first and third strokes and the second and fourth strokes, in order to provide some insights for coaches and players, and further enrich the theory and methods of table tennis match analysis.

2 Method

2.1 Data Samples

10 matches between Japanese table tennis player ITO Mima and Chinese players including Ding Ning, Zhu Yuling, Chen Meng, Liu Shiwen, Wang Manyu and Chen Xingtong in 2018 are taken as samples, as are shown in Table 1.

Table 1. Ten women's table tennis matches of Japanese player ITO Mima

No.	Matches	Opponents	Results
1	4 Nov, Swedish Open, Final	Zhu Yuling	4:0
2	3 Nov, Swedish Open, Semi Final	Ding Ning	4:2
3	3 Nov, Swedish Open, Quarter Final	Liu Shiwen	4:3
4	10 Jun, Japan Open, Final	Wang Manyu	4:2
5	10 Jun, Japan Open, Semi Final	Chen Xingtong	4:3
6	5 May, World Team Championships, Final	Liu Shiwen	3:2
7	2 Jun, China Open, Semi Final	Wang Manyu	1:4
8	26 May, Hong Kong Open, Semi Final	Wang Manyu	3:4
9	24 Mar, German Open, Round Two	Sun Yingsha	3:4
10	25 Feb, Team World Cup, Final	Ding Ning	0:3

Note: No. 1–6 are the matches of ITO Mima won, No. 7–10 are the matches she lost.

2.2   Observation Indices and Collection System

According to the nature of table tennis matches and the stroke types of players, this study took 47 observation indices in 7 categories, including 10 stroke placements, 14 stroke techniques, 4 stroke positions, 6 game actions, 5 stroke effects, 6 stroke spins and 2 stroke results, as is shown in Table 2. On this basis, a table tennis match collection system with three main functions including video monitoring, video editing and technical and tactical information editing was constructed to record the indices and the results of players' last strokes. In addition, based on the nature of the observed indices, this study automatically linked some indices, making manual acquisition more efficient and accurate. For example: (1) when the player used offensive techniques, the ball can only be a long placement on the opponent's table (forehand, middle and backhand); (2) when the ball was in the forehand position, the player could only use the forehand or the pivot position to strike the ball; and when the ball was in the backhand position, the player could only strike the ball with the backhand or backhand turn position; (3) When ITO Mima attacked in the backhand position, the spin of the ball was sink.

The objectivity of the observation indices was confirmed by the agreement of two independent observers by using Cohen's kappa statistics (Inter-Rater-Agreement)

Table 2. Observation indices of table tennis matches

Stroke techniques	Stroke placements	Stroke positions	Game actions	Stroke effects	Stroke spins	Results
Pendulum	Short forehand	Forehand	Serve	Scoring	Strong topspin	Scoring
Reverse	Half long forehand	Backhand	Receive	Better	Normal topspin	Losing
Tomahawk	Long forehand	Pivot	Stalemate	Normal	No spin	
Topspin	Short middle	Backhand turn	Offence	Worse	Strong downspin	
Attack	Half long middle		Defense	Losing	Normal downspin	
Smash	Long middle		Control		Sink	
Flick	Short backhand					
Twist	Half long backhand					
Push	Long backhand					
Touch short	Special					
Slide						
Block						
Lob						
Other						

Note 1: In the category of "stroke technique" in Table 2, "Other" represents unconventional or undistinguishable stroke techniques adopted by players.

Note 2: In the category of "stroke placements" in Table 2, "Special" represents net or edge.

(Robson 2002). The 10 matches including 57 games were selected from the examined games for this purpose. The Cohen's *kappa* values (*k*) of the observation indices were found to be $k = 0.925$ for the "stroke technique", $k = 0.977$ for the "stroke placement", $k = 0.969$ for the "stroke position", $k = 0.966$ for the "game action", $k = 0.989$ for the "stroke effect", $k = 0.915$ for the "stroke spin" and $k = 1$ for the "scoring or losing".

2.3   Multi-dimensional Analytical System

As a natural time series, table tennis match is featured by both players taking turns to strike the ball. Most of the traditional game analysis systems analyze the statistics of a certain stroke or a certain phase, such as the scoring rate and usage rate of the third stroke or the phase of serve and attack, which lacks detailed analysis of tactics composed of two strokes. As a result, coaches and players can only get rough information of the whole match. They cannot know the specific tactics used and the specific technique, placement, position and other information about the tactics without watching the videos. Therefore, this study builds a multi-dimensional analysis system for table tennis matches through data mining algorithms, video interaction and data visualization.

The system can freely choose and combine the starting and ending positions, length, specific attributes of each stroke and types of the tactics. The graphical distribution of their scoring rates and usage rates can be obtained in real time. In addition, after selecting the tactics in which the coaches and players are interested, the system can display the trajectory of the selected tactics on the table and the specific information of each stroke, and provide corresponding video viewing, export and merging, as are shown in Figs. 1 and 2.

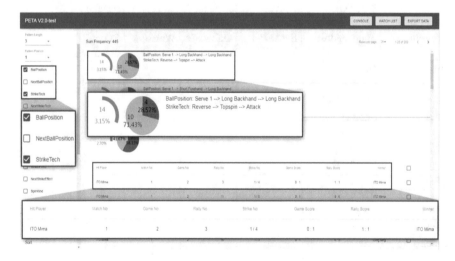

Fig. 1. Multi-dimensional analytical system of table tennis matches (a). Note 1: The box on the left of Fig. 1 includes 7 categories, and researchers can choose one or more of them as analysis samples. Note 2: The box at the top of Fig. 1 includes scoring and usage rates for a specific tactic, as well as times of them. Note 3: The box at the bottom of Fig. 1 includes the number of game, rally, strike, and winner for a specific tactic.

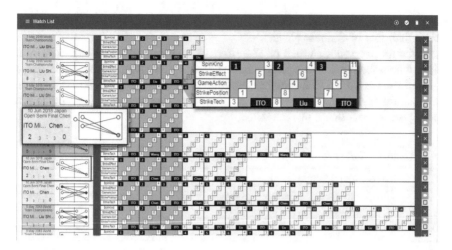

Fig. 2. Multi-dimensional analytical system of table tennis matches (b). Note 1: The box on the left of Fig. 2 includes partial information of the match and the trajectory of the stroke placements on the table. Note 2: The box on the right of Fig. 2 includes the codes of the stroke spin, effect, position, technique and Game action, and each code represents one index.

2.4 Tactics of Serve Round (Stroke 1–3) and Receive Round (Stroke 2–4)

This paper takes the most important indices in table tennis matches – stroke techniques and placements to analyze the tactics of serve round (stroke 1–3) and receive round (stroke 2–4) of ITO Mima (Tang et al. 2010). There are four reasons for that: (1) Serving and receiving are the starting points for using table tennis tactics, and table tennis tactics are composed of one player continuously strike the ball twice (serve as strike once); (2) Techniques and tactics of the first four strokes are the most diverse in table tennis matches, while from the fifth stroke, there are few changes in tactics; (3) Combinations and changes in stroke technique and stroke placement are the cores of table tennis tactics, the former can change stroke spins and game actions by using different techniques, meanwhile, every stroke indices, including stroke technique is also reflected though the latter; (4) The stroke techniques and placements are the most easily observed of 7 categories by researchers.

3 Results

3.1 Basic Data

Table 3 displays the effective tactics which show a scoring rate over 50.0%. In the serve round, 85 types of effective tactics are used by ITO Mima, 6 types more than those adopted by Chinese players, and the total quantities of their tactics are 199 and 163 respectively. However, the mean scoring rate of ITO Mima is 78.4% i.e. 4.4% lower than that of Chinese players. It shows that compared with Chinese players, the effective tactics adopted by ITO Mima in the serve round are more diverse, but less of threats than that of Chinese players.

In the receive round, a total of 134 effective tactics in 100 types are used by ITO Mima, outnumbering Chinese players both in quantity and type. The mean scoring rate of ITO Mima is 90.3%, 0.2% higher than that of Chinese players (90.1%). It can be seen that although the effective tactics of Chinese players barely change, the effective tactics pose a great threat to ITO Mima, too.

Table 3. Basic data of effective tactics between ITO Mima and Chinese players

	Serve round (stroke 1–3)				Receive round (stroke 2–4)			
	Sum	Tactic type	Mean UR	Mean SR	Sum	Tactic type	Mean UR	Mean SR
ITO Mima	199	85	1.18%	78.4%	134	100	1.00%	90.3%
Chinese	163	79	1.27%	82.8%	111	75	1.33%	90.1%

Note: In Table 3, mean UR = (1/tactic type) × 100%. For instance, in the present study, the number of effective tactics for matches in the serving round of ITO Mima was 199, which were of 85 tactic types, then the mean UR was 1.18%, meaning that every tactic was used 2.34 times on average. And mean SR = (scoring tactics/tactic sum) × 100%, meaning that scoring tactics were 156.01 times on average.

3.2   Frequently Used Effective Tactics of ITO Mima

Based on the data of matches, this study defines the frequently used effective tactics of ITO Mima which show a scoring rate over 50.0%, usage rate over 1.5% (serve round) and 1.0% (receive round) respectively and finds out 11 tactics eligibly, as are shown in Tables 4 and 5.

Tactics of the Serve Round. Table 4 presents frequently used effective tactics of ITO Mima. The tactics can be interpreted as follows. For example, "(1) P_A Reverse serve → Short Forehand, P_B Push → Long Backhand, P_A Topspin - - > P_A Scoring" is a frequently used effective tactic in the serve round. It can be understood as "P_A reverse serves the ball to short forehand, P_B returns the ball with a push to long backhand, then P_A strikes the ball with topspin in the third stroke; P_A scores in this rally (the strokes of the rally include P_A scoring the point in the third and other strokes like the 5, 7, or 9 stroke, hereinafter the same)." The usage and scoring rate of this tactic is 2.9% and 53.8%, respectively.

In the serve round, there are 7 frequently used effective tactics. Tactics (2), (3), (4) and (7) are similar to tactic (1), and the latter has the highest usage rate (2.9%), but lowest scoring rate. Tactic (5) has the highest scoring rate (88.9%).

Table 4. Frequently used effective tactics in the serve round of ITO Mima

Serve round tactics (stroke 1–3)	Usage rate (%)	Scoring rate (%)
(1) P_A Reverse serve → Short Forehand, P_B Push → Long Backhand, P_A Topspin - - > P_A Scoring	2.9	53.8
(2) P_A Reverse serve → Short Middle, P_B Push → Long Backhand, P_A Topspin - - > P_A Scoring	2.7	58.3
(3) P_A Reverse serve → Short Backhand, P_B Push → Long Backhand, P_A Topspin - - > P_A Scoring	2.0	55.6
(4) P_A Pendulum serve → Short Middle, P_B Push → Long Backhand, P_A Topspin - - > P_A Scoring	2.0	66.7
(5) P_A Reverse serve → Short Backhand, P_B Touch short → Short Middle, P_A Touch short - - > P_A Scoring	2.0	88.9
(6) P_A Reverse serve → Long Backhand, P_B Topspin → Long Middle, P_A Attack - - > P_A Scoring	1.8	62.5
(7) P_A Pendulum serve → Short Backhand, P_B Push → Long Backhand, P_A Topspin - - > P_A Scoring	1.6	57.1

Note: P_A and P_B represent ITO Mima, Chinese players, respectively

Tactics of the Receive Round. Table 5 presents frequently used effective tactics of ITO Mima. The tactics can be interpreted as another example, "(1) (Long Middle), P_A Attack → Long Backhand, P_B Topspin → Long Backhand, P_A Attack - - > P_A Scoring" is a frequently used effective tactic in the receive round. It can be understood as "(P_B serves the ball to long middle), P_A return the ball with attack to long backhand, then P_B strikes the ball with topspin to long backhand in the third stroke, and P_A strikes the ball with attack in the fourth stroke; P_A Scores in this rally (the strokes of the rally include P_A scoring the point in the fourth and other strokes like the 6, 8, or 10 stroke, hereinafter the same)." The usage and scoring rate of this tactic is 3.2% and 54.5%, respectively.

In the receive round, there are 4 frequently used effective tactics. Tactic (1), (2), (3) and (4) have the same characteristics: P_B serves the ball to long middle (backhand) or half long backhand, P_A return the ball with attack (topspin) to long middle

Table 5. Frequently used effective tactics in the receive round of ITO Mima

Receive round tactics (stroke 2–4)	Usage rate (%)	Scoring rate (%)
(1) (Long Middle), P_A Attack → Long Backhand, P_B Topspin → Long Backhand, P_A Attack - - > P_A Scoring	3.2	54.5
(2) (Long Backhand), P_A Attack → Long Middle, P_B Topspin → Long Forehand, P_A Attack - - > P_A Scoring	1.5	60.0
(3) (Long Backhand), P_A Topspin → Long Middle, P_B Block → Long Backhand, P_A Attack - - > P_A Scoring	1.2	75.0
(4) (Half Long Backhand), P_A Topspin → Long Backhand, P_B Topspin → Long Backhand, P_A Attack - - > P_A Scoring	1.2	75.0

(backhand), then P_B strikes the ball with topspin or block to long backhand (forehand) in the third stroke, and P_A strikes the ball with attack in the fourth stroke. Meanwhile, tactic (1) has the highest usage rate (3.2%), while tactic (3) and (4) have the highest scoring rates.

4 Conclusion

(1) The collection system has three main functions, including video monitoring, video editing, technical and tactical information editing;

(2) Match data, videos and tactical graphics provided by the analytical system can help players and coaches understand tactics more quickly and meticulously;

(3) The effective tactics of ITO Mima are more diverse and aggressive in the receive round; and the main tactic of her is serving the ball to short, and striking with topspin in backhand initiatively (serve round), while in the receive round, attack and topspin in backhand are most obvious technical and tactical features.

(4) The application of data mining and modeling in game analysis can reduce the judgment error by human, and make the results more objective and accurate.

References

Fuchs, M., Liu, R., Lanzoni, I.M., Munivrana, G., Straub, G., Tamaki, S., et al.: Table tennis match analysis: a review. J. Sport. Sci. **36**(23), 2653–2662 (2018)

Tang, J., Cao, H., Deng, Y.: The formation and application of tactic combination model in the table tennis competition. J. Beijing Sport. Univ. **33**(11), 108–110 (2010)

Robson, C.: Real World Research, 2nd edn. Blackwell, Oxford (2002)

Wu, H., Li, Z., Tao, Z., Ding, W., Zhou, J.: Methods of actual strength evaluation and technical diagnosis in table tennis match. J. Natl. Res. Inst. Sport. Sci. **1**, 32–41 (1989)

Yang, Q., Zhang, H.: Application of BP neural network and multiple regression in table tennis technical and tactical ability analysis. J. Chengdu Sport. Univ. **42**(1), 78–82 (2016)

Zhang, H., Yu, L., Hu, J.: Computer-aided game analysis of net sports in preparation of Chinese teams for Beijing Olympics. Int. J. Comput. Sci. Sport. **9**(3), 53–69 (2010)

Zhang, H., Zhou, Z.: An analytical model of the two basic situation strategies in table tennis. Int. J. Perform. Anal. Sport. **17**(6), 970–985 (2017)

Zhang, H., Zhou, Z., Yang, Q.: Match analyses of table tennis in China: a systematic review. J. Sport. Sci. **36**(23), 2663–2674 (2018)

Measurement and Performance Evaluation of Lob Technique Using Aerodynamic Model in Badminton Matches

Lejun Shen[1(✉)], Hui Zhang[2], Min Zhu[1], Jia Zheng[3], and Yawei Ren[1]

[1] Chengdu Sport University, Tiyuan Road, Chengdu, China
sljcool@sina.com
[2] Zhejiang University, Tianmushan Road, Hangzhou, China
zhang_hui@zju.edu.cn
[3] Sichuan Sports College, Taipingsi Road, Chengdu, China
http://www.shenlj.cn/en

Abstract. In badminton matches, lob is a special technique and can be classified into two categories: defensive and offensive. These lobs are difficult to quantitatively measure, analyze, and evaluate. In this paper, we propose a new aerodynamic model to estimate the 3D trajectory from a single camera video and evaluate the performance of lobs. The experimental results show that this model is reliable. Offensive lobs are easily identified by the height of the trajectory. Good lobs are placed farther from the opponent than the bad lobs.

Keywords: Badminton · Computer vision · Ordinary differential equations · Lob · Aerodynamic model · Monocular 3D reconstruction

1 Introduction

Badminton is a popular racket sport included in Olympic Games. In badminton matches, the number of strokes of a rally can vary considerably due to several possible tactical actions. Lob is a special technique because it causes an opponent to move and traverse their defensive space [4]. Lobs can be classified into two categories, namely, defensive and offensive. The offensive lob is a flat trajectory toward the back of the opponent's court, and the defensive lob generates a rising trajectory. These lobs are difficult to quantitatively measure, analyze, and evaluate. Thus, the 3D shuttlecock trajectory is vital in badminton game analysis. In this paper, we propose a new physical model to estimate the 3D trajectory from a single camera video and evaluate the performance of lobs.

In 2017, Shen et al. obtained a 3D ball trajectory from a single-view television video by using a confirming point method and an air-ball friction model [6]. It's hidden assumption is that the air-ball friction coefficient is constant during the flight. Physical theory indicates that a shuttlecock in flight is subject to two

© Springer Nature Switzerland AG 2020
M. Lames et al. (Eds.): IACSS 2019, AISC 1028, pp. 53–58, 2020.
https://doi.org/10.1007/978-3-030-35048-2_7

distinct forces, namely, gravity and air drag force. A natural-feather shuttlecock
is an extremely high-drag projectile. Thus, the air-ball friction coefficient is not
constant, and consequently the 3D trajectory has no analytical solution.

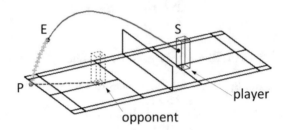

Fig. 1. Offensive lob in badminton game. Please see the text for more details.

The proposed aerodynamic model includes six ordinary differential equations
(ODEs). As shown in Fig. 1, we use these equations to reconstruct the 3D shuttlecock trajectory (red trajectory) and evaluate the placement of lobs (blue dot
P). Given a starting point (S), ending point (E), and flight time t, these ODEs
find the initial velocity vector V_S and consequently reconstruct the 3D trajectory.

Moreover, given S and V_S, these ODEs generate a prolonged (green) 3D trajectory using a very large flight time (e.g., 4 s). The placement can be computed
by the intersection of trajectory and ground plane. The experimental results
show that the reconstructed 3D trajectories are more accurate than those produced by previous models and that the computed placements indicate the quality
of lobs in a badminton match.

1.1 Aerodynamic Model of the Shuttlecock in a Badminton Match

In badminton matches, the human body and shuttlecock must obey physical
rules. For example, the flying shuttlecock (from S to E in Fig. 1) is subject to
two distinct forces: gravity and air drag force. Gravity is a constant force denoted
by g, and air drag force is proportional to the square of the velocity, which is
denoted by

$$f = C_D \frac{1}{2} \frac{\pi d^2}{4} \rho v^2 \tag{1}$$

where C_D is the drag coefficient (=0.59) [1], d is the shuttlecock diameter
(=0.06 m), ρ is the density of air (=1.29 kg/m^3) and v is the velocity. The direction of the drag force is in the exactly opposite direction of velocity. Hence, the
coefficient of air drag acceleration is

$$\alpha = C_D \frac{1}{2} \frac{\pi d^2}{4} \frac{1}{m} \rho \tag{2}$$

Using the above physical model, the motion of shuttlecock can be modeled as the following set of coupled first-order ODEs

$$\frac{\partial x}{\partial t} = v_x$$

$$\frac{\partial y}{\partial t} = v_y$$

$$\frac{\partial z}{\partial t} = v_z$$

$$\frac{\partial v_x}{\partial t} = -\alpha v v_x \tag{3}$$

$$\frac{\partial v_y}{\partial t} = -\alpha v v_y$$

$$\frac{\partial v_z}{\partial t} = -g - \alpha v v_z$$

where (x, y, z) and (v_x, v_y, v_z) denote the position and velocity of the shuttlecock trajectory, v is the velocity $\sqrt{v_x{}^2 + v_y{}^2 + v_z{}^2}$, t is time, g is the acceleration of gravity $(9.8\,\mathrm{m/s^2})$, and α is the coefficient of air drag acceleration $(=0.2152)$.

The above set of equations has no analytical expression. Given a starting point S, initial velocity V_S, and flight time t, these equations simulate a numerical 3D trajectory

$$f_i(S, V_s, t) \tag{4}$$

for i $= 1, 2, 3$. This simulation is a solution of ODSs.

2   Application of Aerodynamic Model to Monocular 3D Reconstruction

Traditional monocular 3D reconstruction methods [5] estimate the 3D trajectory by fitting an analytically expressed physical model in 3D space to observations in 2D images. However, previous ODEs (3) have no analytical expression. Thus, we transform the monocular 3D reconstruction problem into a two-point Boundary Value problem.

First, we obtain the starting point $S = (x_S, y_S, z_S)$ and ending point $E = (x_E, y_E, z_E)$ by using the confirming point method [6]. Second, the flight time t is the duration between the starting and ending point in the video. Given these two points (S and E) and flight time t, the initial velocity $V_S = (V_{x,S}, V_{y,S}, V_{z,S})$ at the starting point S can be computed by a shooting method [3]. Third, the shooting method is a multidimensional root-finding method. The method finds the adjustment of the free parameters V_S to minimize the discrepancy between the ending point E and $f(S, V_S, t)$ to zero

$$x_E - f_1(x_S, y_S, z_S, V_{x,S}, V_{y,S}, V_{z,S}, t) = 0 \tag{5}$$

$$y_E - f_2(x_S, y_S, z_S, V_{x,S}, V_{y,S}, V_{z,S}, t) = 0 \tag{6}$$

$$z_E - f_3(x_S, y_S, z_S, V_{x,S}, V_{y,S}, V_{z,S}, t) = 0 \tag{7}$$

This root-finding problem can be solved by the Newton-Raphson method [3]. The initial guess for the root is the solution of ODEs (3) without air drag force, i.e., $\alpha = 0$. We use a numerical difference to approximate local derivatives because ODEs have no analytical expression. Newton-Raphson method converges quadratically and has one and only one solution.

Table 1. Comparison of different methods.

Method	Smash Speed (m/s)	Mean-Square Error
Gravity model [5]	25.14 ± 4.91	5988.99
Air-ball friction model [6]	–	1559.37
Our aerodynamic model (3)	$\mathbf{96.83 \pm 14.11}$	**179.73**

We build a Hawkeye dataset, in which the smash speed is collected from the television videos. The smash speed of this dataset is $102.39 \pm 4.75\,\mathrm{m/s}$. We also compute the smash speed using different monocular 3D reconstruction methods [5,6]. We then compare the difference between the Hawkeye dataset and two reconstruction methods.

In Table 1, the smaller MSE (Mean-Square Error) indicates the corresponding method is the better. The error of [5] is maximal because it does not consider the air drag force. The error of our aerodynamic model (3) is minimal because they are more realistic than the gravity model [5] or the constant air-ball friction model [6]. This evidence suggests that our method is reliable and the air drag force influences the measurement process significantly and cannot be ignored.

3   Application of Aerodynamic Model to Badminton Technique Evaluation

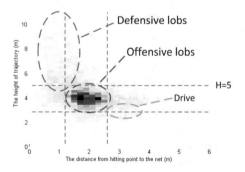

Fig. 2. Difference between defensive and offensive lobs

In racket sports, the placement of strokes is an important factor to achieve the tactical aim. In a badminton match, however, the shuttlecock never lands on the ground except the final stroke. We cannot find the landing area because image evidence is not available; rather, the landing area can only be computed by numerical simulation. Given the starting point S, initial velocity V_S, and flight time t, the 3D trajectory can be represented by a series of line segments computed by the fourth-order Runge-Kutta method [3].

We collected 8,699 strokes from 10 badminton television videos and obtained the players' hitting positions, the opponents' locations, and the shuttlecock's 3D trajectory.

The height of the trajectory (H) is the maximum Z-value of the 3D trajectory, and D is the distance from the hitting point to the net. Figure 2 shows the H-D distribution of lobs. This distribution can be divided into two categories, namely, defensive and offensive lobs, by a horizontal line (H = 5). The majority of lobs are offensive lobs. This result confirms the observation that badminton players are more willing to attack than defend.

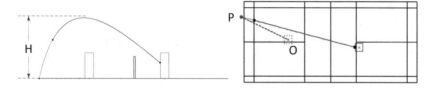

Fig. 3. Height (H) of the trajectory and distance from the placement to the opponent (PO)

Given a very large flight time (e.g., 4 s), ODEs generate a series of line segments (3D trajectory). This 3D trajectory is longer than the true 3D trajectory and intersects the ground plane. The intersection point is called *virtual placement*. In Fig. 3, the blue dotted line PO is the distance from the virtual placement (P) to the opponent (O) gives us a quantitative evaluation of lob technique.

A total of 117 lobs were used by receiving players, Long Chen, to serve; this total included 100 good lobs and 17 bad lobs. Figure 4 shows the distribution of distances from the placement to the opponent. Red rectangles indicate good lobs, while blue rectangles indicate bad lobs. Bad lobs are defined by the opponent's next action and lead to the opponent's smashing and scoring. This result indicates that good lobs are placed farther from the opponent than bad lobs.

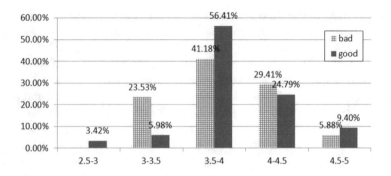

Fig. 4. Distributions of distance from the placement to the opponent (PO)

4   Conclusion

– The shuttlecock motion model presented in this work involves a set of six ODEs. This physical model is highly realistic in badminton games and, consequently, more accurate than traditional models. This model is reliable for evaluating badminton technique. The source code of (3) and the dataset can be found in our home page "http://www.shenlj.cn/en".
– In badminton games, two types of lobs are used, namely, defensive and offensive. Offensive lobs are easily identified by the height of the trajectory using our monocular 3D reconstruction method. Good lobs are placed farther from the opponent than bad lobs based on the distance from the placement to the opponent.
– The proposed shuttlecock motion model helps us both acquire data and analyze badminton games.

References

1. Alam, F., Chowdhury, H., Theppadungporn, C., Subic, A.: Measurements of aerodynamic properties of badminton shuttlecocks. Procedia Eng. **2**, 2487–2492 (2010)
2. Kolbinger, O., Lames, M.: Ball trajectories in tennis - lateral and vertical placement of right handed men's singles serves. Int. J. Perform. Anal. Sport. **13**(3), 750–758 (2013)
3. Press, W.H., Teukolsky, S.A., Flannery, B.P.: Numerical recipes in C (2nd edn.): The Art of Scientific Computing. Cambridge University Press, New York (1992)
4. Ren, Y., Shen, L., Yang, G., Chai, H.: The spacial utility of badminton players in 3D space-games between LIN Dan and Viktor Axelsen. China Sport. Sci. **38**(3), 80–89 (2018)
5. Shen, L., Liu, Q., Li, L., Yue, H.: 3D reconstruction of ball trajectory from a single camera in the ball game International. In: Symposium on Computer Science in Sports (IACSS 2015), pp. 33–39. Springer (2015)
6. Shen, L., Liu, Q., Li, L., Ren, Y.: Reconstruction of 3D ball/shuttle position by two image points from a single view. In: International Symposium on Computer Science in Sport (IACSS 2017), pp. 89–96. Springer (2017)

Applications in Sports Sciences

History of Cybernetics in Sports in the USSR

Models Released in the 1960s

Egor A. Timme[1,2(✉)], Alexander A. Dayal[1,2],
and Yuri A. Kukushkin[2]

[1] Moscow Center of Advanced Sport Technologies (MCAST),
Sovetskoy Armii St. 6, 129272 Moscow, Russia
timme.ea@mossport.ru, alexrhea9999@gmail.com
[2] Russian Association of Computer Science in Sport (RACSS),
Sovetskoy Armii St. 6, 129272 Moscow, Russia
info@racss.ru

Abstract. In this article we provide a review of the emergence and development of Cybernetics in sports in the USSR as well as major events in this field. We also present original mathematical models of sports performance created by Soviet mathematicians and physiologists.

Keywords: History of cybernetics · Soviet researchers in sports science · Mathematical models of sports performance · Cybernetics in sports

1 Introduction

Cybernetics had its origins deep down in the history of science and established long before Cybernetics official appearance and recognition in the world. Cybernetics establishment as a branch of science was due to the whole course of scientific thought development for a long period of time. Paying tribute to the American and European physiologists and mathematicians who took part in the foundation of Cybernetics, such as N. Wiener, W. Ashby, A. Rosenblüth, L. Genderson, C. Bell, C.C. Sherington and others, it is appropriate to mention Russian and Soviet scientists who made a significant contribution to the promotion of Cybernetics as a science, including Cybernetics in sports [1].

1.1 Background and Development of Cybernetics in the USSR

In the 19th century, Russian mathematician I.A. Vyshnegradsky proposed a theory of automatic control via feedback. This theory was the first step in Cybernetics development. A second important step was made by I.P. Pavlov whose physiological concepts of higher nervous system activity and reflexes had a direct impact on the founder of Cybernetics Norbert Wiener. Reflex theory was the prerequisite of the fundamental principle of Cybernetics - regulation by means of feedback. Also, ideas preceding the notion of negative feedback can be found in works of great Russian medical scientist I.M. Sechenov.

© Springer Nature Switzerland AG 2020
M. Lames et al. (Eds.): IACSS 2019, AISC 1028, pp. 61–68, 2020.
https://doi.org/10.1007/978-3-030-35048-2_8

The principle of negative feedback was formulated most closely to the contemporary interpretation by physiologist N.A. Belov in 1925. He formulated this principle on the basis of his own experiments, although his name was forgotten by the physiological community. Long before N. Wiener a more deliberate and thorough definition of this principle was formulated by N.A. Bernstein, founder of the physiology of activity. He introduced the concept of a "reflex ring", realizing insufficiency of the concept of a reflex arc, and gave a detailed structural and functional description of the hierarchical organization of movement control [2].

The pinnacle of Cybernetic is a systemic approach, to which a significant contribution was made by the Soviet physiologist P.K. Anokhin, who developed the theory of functional systems of the body. Such systems are formed depending on the goal [3]. Moreover, V.N. Novoseltsev developed mathematical theory of homeostasis [4]. It is also impossible not to mention the outstanding philosopher A.A. Bogdanov and his monograph "General Organizational Science (Tectology)" which describes the patterns of development of any system, which anticipated many of the provisions of Cybernetics (e.g. feedback principle, control, modeling) [1].

A great contribution to the development of Cybernetics was made by the mathematician A.A. Lyapunov, who was awarded the medal of the International Computer Society "Computer Pioneer" as the founder of Soviet Cybernetics [1]. He created a universal scheme of any complex object, including a living one. This scheme implied the hierarchical decomposition of the vital processes of the organism into elementary parts and processes. He also established several scientific schools in various branches of Cybernetics. The main events of this time was publication in 1958 of the journal "Issues in Cybernetics" edited by A.A. Lyapunov, as well as the organization of a large seminar on Cybernetics at Moscow State University under his leadership. Lyapunov's role in the development of Cybernetics in the USSR was enormous. It was him who was largely responsible for the high level of works in the field of Cybernetics in the USSR [5].

It is also impossible to bypass the contribution of academician G.I. Marchuk, the last President of the USSR Academy of Sciences and the founder of the Institute of Computational Mathematics of the Russian Academy of Sciences. He developed the Cybernetic approach in relation to immunology [6]. In 1959 the Scientific Council on the complex issues of Cybernetics was founded at the Academy of Sciences of the USSR. We owe the appearance of this Council to A. Berg, whose talents as organizer allowed him to overcome all the obstacles on his way [5].

The final step toward implementation of Cybernetics in scientific practice in USSR was publication of N. Wiener's book "Cybernetics" in Russian language for mathematicians, biologists, physiologists, physicians. A new era for Cybernetics in various fields began [7]. In the 1960s and 1970s, cybernetic research in the USSR began to flourish. Cybernetics began to penetrate into all spheres of science and practice, including sports [8, 9].

2   The First Steps of Cybernetics in Sports in the USSR

2.1   Scientific Conferences on the Issues of Cybernetics in Sports

First Conference in 1965. One of the most significant milestones in Cybernetics in sports in the USSR was the hosting of the first USSR Conference "Cybernetics and Sport" on November 1–2, 1965. Conference was devoted to the application of mathematical approaches to the analysis and management of sports activities and took place in Moscow in Soviet Order of Lenin Institute of Physical Education (now, SCOLIPE).

By that time, a large number of attempts were made to apply cybernetic theories to the field of physical activity and sports. However, they were not systematized and interrelated. The conference was attended by 700 people, 120 reports were announced, within 3 days 67 reports were presented [10].

Among the participants of the conference were scientists from the field of biomechanics, biochemistry, morphology and physiology of sport, engineers, specialists in mathematics, as well as trainers, and teachers of physical education. The main areas of the conference were:

- Research and mathematical modeling of physiological processes during muscle activity;
- Simulation of the physical condition in athletes (assessment of fitness);
- Modeling of training processes;
- Simulation of sports activities;
- Methods of collecting and processing data in the process of performing sports exercises.

At the opening ceremony of The Conference, the introductory speech was made by one of the founders of the cybernetic approach in physiology, professor N. A. Bernstein. He talked about the role of cybernetic research in the human motor activity. The Conference participants expressed the unanimous opinion that some attempts are needed to coordinate scientific researches in order to unite discrete research teams in various organizational systems. Systems were ranging from the sports systems to the Academy of Sciences of the USSR and the Allied Academies of Sciences. This plethora of organizations and groups of researchers required special coordinating center.

Such a center was soon established – it was given a very cumbersome and bulky name – popular back those days in USSR - the All-Union Scientific Committee on Cybernetics at the Scientific and Methodological Council of the Union of Sports Societies and Organizations of the USSR.

Second Conference in 1968. The Second Conference "Cybernetics and Sport" was held on the initiative of the abovementioned agency. The section of the Scientific and Methodological Council "Cybernetics and Sport" once again took place in SCOLIPE on September 10–12, 1968. The Conference brought together more than 100 people, representing 39 departments from 27 cities, and 38 oral presentations were made. This conference focused on the following issues:

- General theoretical aspects of the use of computers in sports;
- Multivariate statistical analysis of research results in sports;
- Usage of computers to solve biomedical problems.

To sum up the work of the conference, the chairman professor A.D. Novikov noted the then-growing importance of "mathematization" in scientific research, both in theory and in the practice of sports [11].

2.2   Printed Editions on the Issues of Cybernetics in Sport

In 1969 the first monography on sports Cybernetics was published by V.M. Zatsorsky. In this work he outlined the existing at that time results of the use of cybernetics and mathematics in sports. He also overviewed the methods that have been tested by practitioners [9]. This book played a pivotal role in shaping the outlook of sports scientists in the USSR. In the monthly Soviet journal "Theory and Practice of Physical Culture" a special column "Cybernetics and Sport" was established. Afterwards, the journal began to publish articles on this topic regularly. In 1985, the book "Mathematics and Sport" was published and it immediately gained immense popularity [12].

2.3   The Reverse Side of the Use of Cybernetics in Sports

Despite significant success in mathematical methods in sport, there are still plenty of limitations. In the 1980s, V.M. Zatsorsky wrote that over the past thirty years, mathematical statistics had become universally used in sports science. Unfortunately, even now, there are often a lot of errors and absurdities that this usage leads to the discrediting of statistical methods. There is a tendency towards the emergence of a large number of works that are completely meaningless, or works may contain some major errors, hence, the scientific results are impaired [13].

At the same time, many scientists agreed that it was necessary to make precautions both from underestimating and overestimating the role of the value of Cybernetics and its capabilities in the application to sport. They are also confident that it is impossible to fully replace teachers and coaches by cybernetic tools [10].

3   Models of Sports Performance

At the "Cybernetics and Sport" conferences various methods and models were presented, which were used to analyze data, simulate and manage sports training in various kinds of sports. A special place among them is occupied by models of sports performance, which are applicable to almost all sports. Of particular interest are two models. The first one is based on the representation of biochemical processes under muscular load using kinetic equations. This model was proposed by prominent sports physiologist N.I. Volkov [14, 15].

The second one is based on the mathematical theory of inventory management and methods of calculus of variations. This model was developed by mathematicians, experts in algebra and game theory N.N. Vorobyov, S.S. Kislitsyn and A.S. Mikhailova [16, 17].

3.1 Mathematical Model of Energy Metabolism in Humans During Muscular Activity

Based on facts about the regulation of energy metabolism in a living organism, N.I. Volkov developed kinetic models describing changes in the rate of oxygen consumption and the formation of lactic acid in humans during muscular activity [14, 15]. The models took into account the presence of metabolic autoregulation at the cellular level and the possibility of changing the rate of energy metabolism processes under the influence of various physiological factors associated with diffusion of metabolic products in human body.

Lactic acid is produced in working muscles, enters the heart and then is utilized in the heart, liver, kidneys and non-working muscles throughout the body. Schematically, the system is represented as 6 compartments between flows of varying intensity exist. The model's solution is described as the sum of 6 exponential terms. None of the previous studies of the kinetics of oxygen consumption and lactic acid in humans during muscular activity considered more than two exponential components. Such biexponential dependence is described in a number of papers, and is usually interpreted as the result of the merging of several compartments into a common one.

For muscular work with low intensity, when all oxidative transformations end in the muscles themselves, the process is described by the differential equation:

$$\frac{dx}{dt} = \alpha W - kx \tag{1}$$

For high-intensity work, the process is described by a system of differential Eqs. (2) and (3):

$$\frac{dx_1}{dt} = \alpha W + P_{21} - (k + P_{12})x_1 \tag{2}$$

$$\frac{dx_2}{dt} = P_{12}x_1 - P_{21}x_2 \tag{3}$$

where x_i - concentration of metabolic products and metabolites in blood and tissues, P_{ij} - transfer constants, W - power of work, α - proportionality constant which connects the amount of work with the amount of exchange products, k - oxidation rate constant.

Kinetic models imply an exponential increase in the rate of oxygen consumption and the production of lactic acid during the exercise until reaching a stationary mode of operation. Such models also imply an exponential slowdown of these processes after the end of muscle activity.

These models were the prototype of the development of a well-known and actively used 3-component model of human bioenergy by R.H. Norton. He mentions Volkov's models in his papers [18–20]. Based on these models, a method for determining the quantitative glycolysis parameters describing the biokinetics of endogenous lactate was developed. This method allows determining lactate contribution to the energy supply of sports distances for skaters and rowers [21]. It gives the best results for exercises of a duration from 2 to 4 min, which corresponds to distances of 500 and 1000 m in rowing in canoes.

Limitations of the Models. A comparison was made of the main conclusions of the kinetic models with the results obtained experimentally under various conditions. In some cases, the dynamics of lactic acid in the blood reveals significant oscillatory changes, superimposed on the main course of the "accumulation - elimination" curve of lactic acid. The likelihood of oscillatory changes in the acid curve increases with increasing power of the exercise. This suggests that the presence of oscillation is due to some reasons not taken into account in the model. Among such reasons may be features of the circulation and the behavior of intracellular metabolic systems during intense muscular activity.

3.2   Mathematical Model of Fatigue and Rest

At the First Conference, mathematician Sergey Kislitsyn presented a mathematical model developed in 1961–62 at the Steklov Institute of Mathematics. This model described the processes of fatigue and rest during muscular work, hence, the model was called "fatigue-rest" [16]. This model is based on the theory of inventory management, developed in the works of Bellman, and uses the analogy between the dynamics of stock changes and labor (sports) human activity.

The model assumes that the state of the system (here, the human body) at time t is characterized by a positive number $x(t)$ - the level of working capacity, - included between 0 and 1. Two monotonic functions are set. $g_1(t)$ is the function of decrement in working capacity on a full power and the initial state is set at 1. $h_0(t)$ is the working capacity recovery curve during the rest and the initial state is set at 0. At each time point, two extreme types of behavior are possible: full power work and complete rest. The further course of the change in working capacity is characterized by shifts in the functions g_1 and h_0 (4).

$$g_x(s) = \left(g_1^{-1}(x) + s\right) \qquad h_x(s) = \left(h_1^{-1}(x) + s\right) \tag{4}$$

Intermediate types of behavior are possible, which are described by differential Eq. (5).

$$\dot{x}(t) = \alpha(t)\dot{g}_x(0) + (1 - \alpha(t))\dot{h}_x(0) \tag{5}$$

The resulting work in the interval from t_1 to t_2 is represented by the formula (6).

$$\int_{t_1}^{t_2} \alpha(t)x(t)dt \tag{6}$$

The task is to find a mode that maximizes work for a period of time with a known initial state $x(0)$. Of considerable interest is also the dual task - finding the optimal mode when performing a specific motor task. The study of these problems is reduced to solving problems of the calculus of variations with constraints.

The investigation on this model showed that the optimal behavior largely depends on the so-called value function of the level $r(x)$ $(0 \leq r(x) < x)$, equal to the amount of work per unit of time in the constant mode level x. If $r(x)$ has only one maximum at the point $x = x_0$, then the optimal behavior of the system is that it in the fastest way possible enters the stationary mode. At the same time, system arrives in such mode within a certain time and finishes work in the maximum output mode. It's needed in order to reach the level of $r(x_0)$ at the end of the period.

This qualitative conclusion is consistent with the results of the analysis of the well-known Keller model developed for running [22, 23]. Remarkably, this conclusion was obtained earlier and in a more general form.

Limitations of the Models. The most unrealistic feature of the described model is its non-inertia character. It is natural to assume that the course of the change in the state of the system after the moment t is determined not only by the value of $x(t)$, but also by the previous states (for example, at the beginning of work there is a period of pre-work). Another drawback of the model is the identification of the state of the system, which is multidimensional with a scalar quantity.

4 Conclusion

As a result of the successful development of Cybernetics as a science in the Soviet Union, a breakthrough was made in the development of cybernetic methods in sports in the 1960s and 1980s. Many theories, methods and models made up at that time were included in the world collection of scientific results. These works have not only historical value, but also could be applied now. Unfortunately, some others remained only on the shelves of libraries. Each of these endeavors provided a methodological and technical basis for the successful advancement of Soviet sports science and consequently became one of the main factors for the success of Soviet athletes in the international arena.

Currently, the process of formation and integration of Russian communities in the field of computer science into the global system of scientific and social communications is going on [24]. In this regard, previous successes and traditions play an important role in the process, as well as the hosting the 12th IACSS-2019 Symposium in Russia.

References

1. Fedorov, V.I.: Physiology and Cybernetics: the History of mutual penetration of ideas, modern state and prospects. For the 60th anniversary of the writing of N. Wiener's book "Cybernetics". Successes Physiol. Sci. **38**, 72–86 (2007). (in Russian)
2. Bernstein, N.A.: New lines of development in physiology and their correlation with Cybernetics. In: Philosophical Issues of Physiology of Higher Nervous Activity and Psychology, pp. 299–322 Publishing House of the USSR Academy of Sciences in Moscow (1963). (Russian)
3. Anokhin, P.K.: Cybernetics of functional systems: selected works. Medicine, Moscow (1998). (in Russian)

4. Novoseltsev, V.N.: Control Theory and Biosystems. Analysis of Contractive Features. Nauka, Moscow (1978) (in Russian)
5. Pospelov, D.A.: Formation of Informatics in Russia. In: Pospelov, D.A., Fet, Y.I. (eds.) Essays on the History of Informatics in Russia, pp. 7–44. Scientific Publishing Center UIGGM, Novosibirsk (1998). (in Russian)
6. Marchuk, G.I.: Some mathematical models in immunology. In: Stoer, J. (ed.) Optimization Techniques Part 1, pp. 41–62. Springer, Heidelberg (1978)
7. Viner, N.: Cybernetics or control and connection in animal and machine. Sov. Radio, Moscow (1968). (in Russian)
8. Novikov, D.A.: Cybernetics: From Past to Future. Springer, Heidelberg (2016)
9. Zatsiorsky, V.M.: Cybernetics, mathematics, sports (application of mathematical and cybernetic methods in sports science and in sports practice). Physical Culture and Sport Moscow (1969). (in Russian)
10. Novikov, A.D.: The beginning is made (cybernetics and sports). Theory Pract. Phys. Cult. 11–12 (1966). (in Russian)
11. Smirnov, Y.V.: Cibernetics in sports. Theory Pract. Phys. Cult. 78–80 (1968). (in Russian)
12. Sadovsky, L.E., Sadovsky, A.L.: Mathematics and Sports. Nauka, Moscow (1985). (in Russian)
13. Zatsiorsky, V.M.: Warning: statistics! Theory Pract. Phys. Cult. 52–55 (1989). (in Russian)
14. Volkov, N.I.: The creation of a mathematical model of the processes of energy metabolism during muscular activity. Theory Pract. Phys. Cult. 5, 37–43 (1966). (in Russian)
15. Volkov, N.I.: Mathematical modeling of human energy metabolism in muscle activity. In: Proceedings of the Scientific Conference "Cybernetics and sport", pp. 12–13. SCOLIPE, Moscow (1965). (in Russian)
16. Kislitsyn, F.S., Mikhaylova, A.S., Vorobyev, N.N.: A fatigue-rest model (Optimal behavior of fatigue-rest model). News USSR Acad. Sci. Tech. Cybern. 27–37 (1965). (in Russian)
17. Kislitsyn, F.S.: Principles of mathematical modeling of fatigue and rest. In: Proceedings of the scientific conference "Cybernetics and sport", pp. 13–15. SCOLIPE, Moscow (1965). (in Russian)
18. Morton, R.H.: On a model of human bioenergetics. Eur. J. Appl. Physiol. Occup. Physiol. 54, 285–290 (1985)
19. Morton, R.H.: A three component model of human bioenergetics. J. Math. Biol. 24, 451–466 (1986)
20. Morton, R.H., Gass, G.C.: A systems model approach to the ventilatory anaerobic threshold. Eur. J. Appl. Physiol. Occup. Physiol. 56, 367–373 (1987)
21. Shkumatov, L.M., Moroz, E.A.: Pharmacokinetics of lactate as a primary method of assessing the contribution of anaerobic glycolysis to the energy load in skaters and rowers. In: All-Russian Scientific-Practical Conference with International Participation "Methods of Assessing and Improving Performance in Athletes", pp. 117–119. North-Western State Medical University named after I. I. Mechnikov, Saint-Petersburg (2013). (in Russian)
22. Keller, J.B.: Optimal velocity in a race. Am. Math. Mon. 81, 474–480 (1974)
23. Keller, J.B.: A theory of competitive running. Phys. Today 26, 43 (1973)
24. Timme, E.A., Bogomolov, A.V.: Scientific communications in sports Informatics. Sport. Pedagog. Educ. 183–191 (2018). (in Russian)

Training Plans Optimization Using Approximation and Visualization of Pareto Frontier

Egor A. Timme[1,2(✉)], Alexander A. Dayal[1,2],
and Yuri A. Kukushkin[2]

[1] Moscow Center of Advanced Sport Technologies (MCAST),
Sovetskoy Armii Street 6, 129272 Moscow, Russia
timme.ea@mossport.ru, alexrhea9999@gmail.com
[2] Russian Association of Computer Science in Sport (RACSS),
Sovetskoy Armii Street 6, 129272 Moscow, Russia
info@racss.ru

Abstract. The article presents an approach to the formation of optimal training plans, based on models of performance depending on the training effects and the method of multidimensional multi-criteria optimization - approximation and visualization of the Pareto frontier.

Keywords: Multi-criteria optimization · Optimal training planning · Pareto frontier · Sport performance · Mathematical modelling in sports

1 Introduction

Construction of optimal training load plan in order to achieve the best sports results is one of the most important and intricate tasks of sports theory and practice. The dynamics of the growth of sports results is determined by the specific individual adaptation reactions of the athlete's body to physical activity and, therefore, can be described using mathematical models.

When a coach makes a training plan for an athlete, he/she aims at finding a general solution, while pursuing several additional goals and evaluating possible outcomes, using several criteria. Primarily, a given coach aims to optimize results for a certain competitive day, e.g. using different tapering strategies. At the same time, a coach wants to minimize the total amount of training load for a period of preparation. Obviously, these goals are antagonistic in nature. In order to obtain an increase in the result, the training volume must be increased. At the same time, reducing the amount of physical activity leads to a decrement in the result. Also, if the athlete's body is overloaded, fatigue state occurs, and it also leads to decrease in results. Hence these two goals cannot be achieved at the same time and a compromise between these goals is necessary [1].

The current study offers an approach to optimization of sports results based on one of the methods of multidimensional multi-criteria optimization - approximation and visualization of the Pareto frontier. The method described in this paper consists of

© Springer Nature Switzerland AG 2020
M. Lames et al. (Eds.): IACSS 2019, AISC 1028, pp. 69–76, 2020.
https://doi.org/10.1007/978-3-030-35048-2_9

searching for and visualizing the boundaries of the set of approachability of these two goals, i.e. the Pareto frontier and its demonstration to decision maker, namely, the coach. A coach, pursuing this method, can choose the most preferred training plan.

2 Related Works

There are several types of tasks associated with analyzing the relationship between training loads and performance using mathematical models:

- *Structural identification of the model* - the choice of the type of the model. To describe the relationship between training loads and sports results, both linear and nonlinear parametric models in continuous and discrete forms are used. These models are with constant and variable time parameters characterizing the athlete's adaptation profile [2–6].
- *Parametric identification of the model* - selection of the model parameters according to the data of training loads and tests. Various methods are used to solve this problem—least squares method, maximum likelihood, as well as other recursive methods for time-varying parameters, which are described elsewhere [7–9].
- *Simulation modeling* - calculation of sports performance using a model along with athlete's adaptation profile—i.e. a set of model parameters and a complete exercise plan for training loads [2, 10].
- *Optimization of the training plan* - finding a family of optimal training plans according to certain criteria of training strategies [11–13].

The latter task is the most difficult and laborious one of the abovementioned. The simplest possible and at the same time the most limited approach to its solution is the usage of the classical linear model of Calvert and Banister [2] based on the analysis of influence curves, which is described in the Fitz-Clarke, Morton and Banister study [11].

Schaefer, Asteroth and Ludwig [13] implemented a variety of optimization algorithms to generate optimal training plans for models developed by Banister [2] and Perl [4]. These models are based on finding the maximum of a single objective function (according to one criterion), and other conditions, such as microcycles, off-weeks, days for rest, maximum loads, which were considered as constraints. Finally, the quality of the resulting solutions was evaluated.

The task of performance optimization for small periods during a short taper period for a model with variable parameters was attempted to solve in the work of Thomas and Busso [14]. The optimization approach for the nonlinear model was considered in Turner, Mazzoleni et al. [6]. Articles in which evolutionary algorithms were used to optimize training plans with regard to physiological constraints are given in the works of Kumyaito, Yupapin and others [15, 16].

2.1 Multi-criteria Optimization

Principles of multi-criteria optimization are significantly different from conventional optimization. In the case of one criterion, the goal of problem solving is to find a global solution that gives the minimum or maximum value for a single objective function.

In the case of several criteria, we have several objective functions, each of which can have an optimal value with its own set of values of independent variables.

If the optimal solutions for various objective functions are substantially different, then we can not argue that the optimal solution of the whole problem was found. In this case, we get a set of solutions, none of which is optimal in comparison with the others in all senses (that is, according to all criteria).

2.2 Approaches for Solving Multi-criteria Optimization Problems

In the multi-criteria optimization problem, the m-dimensional vector of values of criteria f is given by the mapping from the space of the system *state Rn* to the linear normalized space of goals (or criteria) R_m: $f = F(x)$.

The desire to achieve several goals at once, which is characteristic if we state multi-criteria problems, leads to a contradiction that can be resolved either by reducing the multi-criteria problem to a single criterion problem by achieving some kind of compromise, or by generalizing the very concept of optimality.

Method of Achievable Goals. Instead of optimal solutions, it is proposed to look for so-called effective solutions, i.e. those that cannot be improved in all criteria simultaneously. Among all the achievable goals, we can emphasize a set of so-called unimprovable goals, i.e. it is impossible to improve the value of one of the criteria without deteriorating the value of the other. A set of unimprovable goals, called a noninferior, or effective set (as well as Edgeworth-Pareto set), is geometrically represented as part of the boundary of the set of achievable goals.

It visually characterizes the sum of compromises that are reasonable from the standpoint of interests under consideration. The method of achievable goals (MAG) allows to receive information about reasonable trade-offs not only between two criteria, but also between three, four or a larger number of criteria.

In the general case of an arbitrary number of criteria, the Edgeworth – Pareto box (EPB) of the set of achievable goals is usually called the sum (or set) of achievable goals, completed with all the criterion points dominated by them. MAG allows to study reasonable compromises based on the study of interconnectedness (objective replacement curves) between non-dominated combinations of criteria values, that is used to assess the quality of a solution [17].

The main steps of MAG are:

(1) the construction of a set of achievable goals (or its EPB) in the space of criteria, i.e. those combinations of criteria values that can be obtained with possible solutions;
(2) a visual study of the set of achievable goals, and especially its effective boundaries (the so-called objective replacement curves between different pairs of criteria);
(3) the choice of the preferred achievable goal of an achievable combination of criteria values;
(4) calculation and visualization of the solution, which will lead to the selected goal [18].

2.3   Pareto Optimality

For a multi-criteria case, the concepts of Pareto-dominance and Pareto-optimality are of importance. The main idea of Pareto optimality is the impossibility of improving the solution according to one of the criteria without deteriorating by the other one [19].

The solution of the multi-criteria optimization problem is the Pareto set $S \subset \Omega$ of all Pareto-optimal permissible points, i.e. such ones that are not dominated by any other valid points. The Pareto set S corresponds to the Pareto frontier $P = F(S)$ (the image of the Pareto-set in the space of objective functions) (Fig. 1). Hence, unlike the single-criterion problem, the answer is not one point, but a set of points. In the Pareto set, the points are not comparable with each other, i.e. all solutions to the problem are equal.

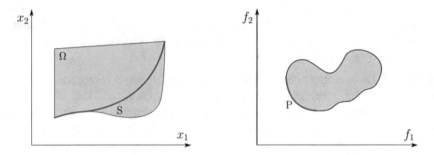

Fig. 1. Pareto set $S \subset \Omega$ in the parameters space (x_1, x_2) and the Pareto frontier $P = f(S)$ in the space of objective functions (f_1, f_2).

2.4   Tradeoff Indicators

As a formal indicator that can be used during comparison of two points on the Pareto frontier, an objective tradeoff between these points (OT) is used, which is defined as:

$$OT(x_1, x_2) = \frac{f_2(x_2) - f_2(x_1)}{f_1(x_2) - f_1(x_1)} \quad (1)$$

This indicator characterizes the "cost" of approaching the target according to one criterion due to another criterion. If we bring the Pareto frontier closer with a continuous regression function, then it makes sense to consider such an indicator as the tradeoff rate (TR):

$$TR(x_0) = \frac{df_1(x_0)}{df_2(x_0)} \quad (2)$$

which is a tangent to the Pareto frontier at x_0 point.

3 Training Plan Optimization

3.1 The Model Used

It makes sense to postulate an optimization problem only for models with constant parameters. The linear classical model [2] describes the phenomena of supercompensation and the plateau effect sufficiently good, but the drawback is that the set of achievability of a sports result is unlimited, i.e. with an increase in the load level the result grows without limit [13]. That is certainly impossible.

This disadvantage is covered by the nonlinear model (2), which is described by a system of differential equations in continuous time [6].

$$\frac{dg}{dt} + \frac{1}{\tau_1} g^\alpha = k_1 w(t) \tag{3}$$

$$\frac{dh}{dt} + \frac{1}{\tau_2} h^\beta = k_2 w(t) \tag{4}$$

$$p(t) = p(0) + g(t) - h(t) \tag{5}$$

where $p(0)$, $p(t)$ are the values of the sports performance at the initial moment and at the moment of time t, respectively; τ_1, τ_2 are the characteristic delay time of the training effect and fatigue, respectively; k_1, k_2 are coefficients of linear effects superposition of exercise and fatigue, respectively. $w(t)$ is the value of the training impulse at the moment of time t; α, β are coefficients that characterize the nonlinearity of the model. When $\alpha = \beta = 1$, this model transforms into the classical Banister linear model [2].

3.2 Models Parameters Values

For numerical experiments with the model (3–5), we took the values of the parameters from previous works [6], which are presented in Table 1.

Table 1. Parameter values and initial conditions for simulations in examples

Parameter	Value
τ_1	70
τ_2	6.5
α	1.18
β	0.96
k_1	0.1
k_2	0.16
p_0	160
f_0	70
g_0	20

3.3   Examples

Linear Model. Approximations of the Pareto frontier for a linear model with non-linearity parameters $\alpha = \beta = 1$ are constructed. Numerical experiments show that the Pareto frontier, when using this model, is a linear function that shifts indefinitely during subsequent iterations in the northeast direction during error set.

Nonlinear Model. Approximation of the Pareto frontier for the nonlinear model (3–5) with the parameter values in Table 1 is shown in Fig. 2.

Also for visualization purposes, there are several arbitrary solutions from the achievable set. A pair of solutions was selected that lie on the Pareto frontier. Training plans for all strategies were generated and the corresponding sports performances were shown. The TR graph corresponding to the Pareto frontier is shown and the OT index between the two selected solutions lying on the boundary is calculated (Table 2).

Table 2. Several training plan comparison and selection of most optimal one

Training plan	Performance	Training volume	Tradeoff rate
1	217.6	1402	0.009
2	233.5	3666	0.017

Objective tradeoff (OT) values between plans 1 and 2, lying on the Pareto frontier, index OT = 0.07.

The second training plan leads to an increase in sports result by 7% more compared to the first, but the cost for this gain is significant - we have to increase the total amount of training load almost 2.6 times.

This example illustrates the approach that is closest to the decision-making when creating the training plan for the period when it is necessary to repeatedly compare the different solutions, choosing the most appropriate according to various criteria the decision.

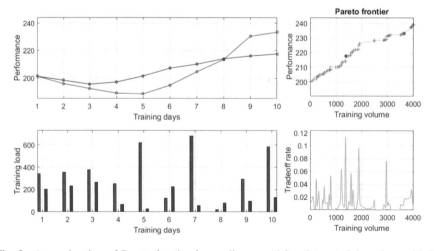

Fig. 2. Approximation of Pareto frontier for nonlinear model and two training plans with its respective performance and tradeoff rate graphs.

4 Discussion

Since we are not dealing with the Pareto frontier itself, but with its approximation with a certain accuracy, it should be noted that different strategies for implementing the search algorithm can produce different approximations.

In the monograph [20] it is shown that the Pareto frontier is unstable, i.e. when small changes in the model parameters are given, the Pareto frontier and its approximation can change significantly.

If the number of criteria is more than two, then the set of achievable goals as well as its non-dominated frontier cannot be depicted as flat figures. In the case of three criteria, the Pareto-frontier is usually a surface that is part of the boundary of the three-dimensional set.

At the same time, MAG allows to find relatively simple forms of representation of the non-dominated set, which are similar in many respects to ordinary geographic maps. Hence, in order to understand the set of achievable goals and the relationships between the criteria, it is necessary to look for ways to visualize it. One of such ways is depiction of sets of two-dimensional sections of a set of achievable goals. In the case of three criteria, a two-dimensional section is understood as the combination of the values of the two criteria that are achievable with a certain fixed value of the third [18, 20].

5 Conclusions

The proposed algorithm for finding Pareto-optimal training plans according to a set of specified criteria allows us to narrow down the space of possible decisions and provides an opportunity for coaches to make a subjective choice taking into account his preferences.

References

1. Timme, E.A.: Optimization of training plans. In: All-Russian Scientific and Practical Conference on Sports Science in Children's and Youth Sports and High Performance Sports, 30 November–2 December 2016. Collection of Materials, pp. 222–225. MCAST, Moscow (2016). (in Russian)
2. Calvert, T.W., Banister, E.W., Savage, M.V., Bach, T.: A systems model of the effects of training on physical performance. IEEE Trans. Syst. Man Cybern. **6**(2), 94–102 (1976)
3. Busso, T., Candau, R., Lacour, J.R.: Fatigue and fitness modelled from the effects of training on performance. Eur. J. Appl. Physiol. **69**, 50–54 (1994)
4. Perl, J.: PerPot: a metamodel for simulation of load performance interaction. Eur. J. Sport Sci. **1**, 1–13 (2001)
5. Busso, T.: From an indirect response pharmacodynamic model towards a secondary signal model of dose-response relationship between exercise training and physical performance. Sci. Rep. **7**, 40422 (2017)
6. Turner, J.D., Mazzoleni, M.J., Little, J.A., Sequeira, D., Mann, B.P.: A nonlinear model for the characterization and optimization of athletic training and performance. Biomed. Hum. Kinet. **9**, 82–93 (2017)

7. http://or.nsfc.gov.cn/bitstream/00001903-5/422669/1/1000014250749.pdf
8. Ljung, L., Soederstroem, T.: Theory and Practice of Recursive Identification. Signal Processing, Optimization, and Control. The MIT Press, Cambridge (1983)
9. Busso, T., Denis, C., Bonnefoy, R., Geyssant, A., Lacour, J.R.: Modeling of adaptations to physical training by using a recursive least squares algorithm. J. Appl. Physiol. (1985) **82**, 1685–1693 (1997)
10. Busso, T., Carasso, C., Lacour, J.R.: Adequacy of a systems structure in the modeling of training effects on performance. J. Appl. Physiol. **71**(5), 2044–2049 (1991)
11. Fitz-Clarke, J.R., Morton, R.H., Banister, E.W.: Optimizing athletic performance by influence curves. J. Appl. Physiol. **71**, 1151–1158 (1991)
12. Thomas, L., Mujika, I., Busso, T.: A model study of optimal training reduction during pre-event taper in elite swimmers. J. Sports Sci. **26**, 643–652 (2008)
13. Schaefer, D., Asteroth, A., Ludwig, M.: Training plan evolution based on training models. In: International Symposium Innovations in Intelligent Systems and Applications (INISTA), Madrid, pp. 1–8. IEEE (2015)
14. Thomas, L., Busso, T.: A theoretical study of taper characteristics to optimize performance. Med. Sci. Sports Exerc. **37**, 1615–1621 (2005)
15. Kumyaito, N., Yupapin, P., Kreangsak, T.: Personalized sports training plans with physiological constraints using the ε-constraint method with a genetic algorithm. Far East J. Electron. Commun. **17**, 475–496 (2017)
16. Kumyaito, N., Yupapin, P., Tamee, K.: Planning a sports training program using Adaptive Particle Swarm Optimization with emphasis on physiological constraints. BMC Res. Notes **11**, 9 (2018)
17. Lotov, A., Bushenkov, V.A., Kamenev, G.K., O.L., C.: Computer and compromise. In: Method of Achievable Goals. Nauka, Moscow (1997). (in Russian)
18. Lotov, A.V., Miettinen, K.: Visualizing the Pareto frontier. In: Multiobjective Optimization, pp. 213–243. Springer, Heidelberg (2008)
19. Podinovskii, V.V., Nogin, V.D.: Pareto-Optimal Solutions of Multicriteria Problems. Nauka, Moscow (1982). (in Russian)
20. Lotov, A.V., Bushenkov, V.A., Kamenev, G.K.: Interactive Decision Maps: Approximation and Visualization of Pareto Frontier. Springer, Boston (2013)

Train4U - Mobile Sport Diagnostic Expert System for User-Adaptive Training

Ingolf Waßmann, Nikolaj Troels Graf von Malotky[✉],
and Alke Martens

University of Rostock, Albert-Einstein-Str. 22, 18059 Rostock, Germany
nikolaj.graf_von_malotky@uni-rostock.de

Abstract. As training plans of athletes are static and are not adapted dynamically towards current conditions (e.g. lack of sleep, hunger, weather, and stress), this contribution depicts an expert system to close this gap. Based on an extensive literature research, relevant parameters that influence sport performance, and explicit effects in the form of rules are detected. An empirical study that we conducted with more than 100 athletes revealed significance levels of certain parameters and further rules. Taking into account this data, a prototype Android application using a rule-based expert system is presented. While some parameters such as weather and location are determined automatically, the remaining parameters are collected by self-assessment that users have to do before and after the workout. All data (also including sensor data during workout) is stored in a database. In future, machine learning technologies will be included in order to derive new rules based on user statistics.

Keywords: Expert system · Virtual coach · Training adaption ·
Sport diagnostic · Empirical study

1 Introduction

In the field of competitive and professional sports, regular performance and fitness tests are conducted in order to evaluate the success of training, to optimize training programs and to give general information about the performance ability during sport activities. In these tests, persons are regularly exposed to physical stress while different physiological parameters are determined, e.g. using lactate diagnostics or spiroergometry. These methods have some disadvantages. Measurements are not performed during real exercises, but under controlled laboratory conditions. Hence, the significance of derived parameters is questionable. Furthermore, measurements are extensive (e.g. spiroergometry) and/or invasive (e.g. lactate diagnostics). Important parameters like oxygen saturation are determined only indirectly. Moreover, these parameters are interesting for amateur sportsmen as they are related to health questions. In this paper, the investigations started with amateur sportsmen as the basis for our empirical study. This is due to the fact that the number of professional sportsmen for one sports area was not available for our research.

Based on near-infrared spectroscopy (NIRS) (Jha 2010), a joint project between the University of Rostock, the University of Wismar, and OXY4 GmbH develops the

© Springer Nature Switzerland AG 2020
M. Lames et al. (Eds.): IACSS 2019, AISC 1028, pp. 77–85, 2020.
https://doi.org/10.1007/978-3-030-35048-2_10

so-called TrainOXY™ system that is designed for application in real sport situations. The mobile solution consists of a small sensor unit that can be attached to any part of the body, and a mobile app for smartphones and smartwatches. This allows non-invasive and real-time monitoring of different parameters like pulse rate (PR), pulse index (PI), tissue hemoglobin index (THI), and muscle oxygen saturation (SmO2) during training sessions. In the sub-project Train4U, the University of Rostock develops an expert system to reveal user-adapted training information based on different parameters that are presented in this contribution. Training plans are generally static, that means once the plan has been created, there's no adaption to current conditions at runtime and the training goal cannot be changed. Parameters like sick days, poor nutrition, lack of sleep, and stress are ignored. Consequently, training goals are not achieved and athletes or coaches cannot take corrective action in time or rather understand the reasons for failure, although appropriate expert knowledge is available. For this reason, we present an approach for monitoring those parameters in order to automatically analyze and optimize current training processes. As a first step, we design a solution targeting amateur sports in order to address a bigger number of users. In future, we will conduct empirical studies with this target group using our application and take the findings to extend our solution for professional sports.

2   Performance Parameters

In order to design an expert system as the foundation of a "virtual coach", it's necessary to determine parameters that influence individual's sport performance. Mental variables play an important role for success in sport, including psychology, sociology, intelligence and creativity (Birrer and Levine 1987). In addition to these internal parameters there are "external factors such as playing environment, voluntary alcohol usage, sleep, emotions, and the team environment" (Dahl 2013). Based on an extensive literature review, we found essential parameters that influence sport performance:

- **internal parameters:**
  - *somatype*: endomorph, mesomorph and ectomorph: (Chaouachi et al. 2005);
  - *talent*: genetic predispositions (Phillips et al. 2010);
  - *age*: child, teenager, middle age, senior (Ericsson 1990; McPherson and Thomas 1989);
  - *psyche*: anger, depression, motivation, etc. (Raglin 2001; Williams 1993);
  - *nutrition*: protein, fat, carbs, minerals, vitamins (Williams 1999);
  - *technique*: sport theory, embodiment (Myer et al. 2011);
  - *sleep*: duration, depth (Savis 1994);
  - *training partner*: mutual motivation and support (Butt et al. 2010);
  - *injury*: temporal physical impairment (Nippert and Smith 2008);
  - *disease*: cold, allergies, etc. (Raglin 2001);
  - *alcohol consumption*: last consumed, quantity (Shirreffs and Maughan 2006);
  - *supplements*: e.g. creatine, caffeine (Williams 2005);
  - *received perception of exertion (RPE)* (Borg 1982);
  - *weather sensitivity*: e.g. weather pain in arthritis (Vihma 2010)

- **external Parameters:**
  - *training time*: morning, after lunch, midnight, etc. (Reilly et al. 2000; Atkinson and Reilly 1996);
  - *training duration*: e.g. sprint vs. marathon (Borresen and Lambert 2009);
  - *environment*: gym, outdoor, synthetic, etc. (Andersson et al. 2008; Kenney et al. 2015);
  - *sports equipment*: quality, protectors, etc. (Timmerman et al. 2015);
  - *weather*: rain, sun, snow, etc. (Vihma 2010; Thornes 1977);
  - *temperature*: heat, cold (Siegel and Laursen 2012; Lindberg et al. 2012);
  - *time of year*: spring, summer, fall, winter (Reilly et al. 2000; Komarow and Postolache 2005).

Considering the found parameters, we developed a questionnaire to determine which parameters have subjective importance for people. Be aware that we are currently working with amateur sportsmen, which we found at the University (e.g. Department of Sports) and in sport clubs in Rostock. For this, test subjects had to rate each of the 21 parameters on a five-point Likert scale: very negative (−1.0), negative (−0.5), no effect (0), positive (0.5), and very positive (1.0). In total, 108 participants took part in the empirical study; eight with missing data so that 100 people have been selected for evaluation (see statistical data in Table 1). 78% of this group affirmed the question if they would call themselves "athletes", doing sports on a regular basis (several times a week).

Table 1. Questionnaire participants

	Men	Women
Participants	63	37
Athletes	49	29
Age	27 ± 11 yrs.	26 ± 22 yrs.
Height	1.82 ± 0.10 m	1.69 ± 0.14 m
Weight	82.5 ± 12 kg	65.5 ± 10 kg
BMI	24.8 ± 5	22.8 ± 5

Analysis of the raw data revealed, that while injury, disease and alcohol consumption have only negative influence on sport performance, the remaining parameters have both negative and positive effects. Figure 1 visualizes the normalized average parameter ratings. Assuming a threshold value of 0.5 (orange line in Fig. 1), most subjective relevant sport performance parameters are nutrition, sleep, training partner, injury, and disease.

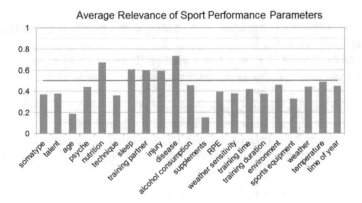

Fig. 1. Normalized average ratings of sport performance parameters

3 Our Expert System Model

Since the TrainOXY™ system is developed for mobile usage (including small, easy to attach sensors, and a mobile app for Android), our virtual coach is subject to the requirements and challenges of human-computer interaction design for mobile devices (Huang 2009) (Harrison, Flood, & Duce 2013). Therefore, it's important to minimize cognitive load of our application so that the primary task – the workout – is not adversely affected. Consequently, we decided to reduce the above-mentioned parameters to an acceptable level in order to minimize user interactions and time consumed. 10 s needed to fill out the form seemed the limit. At a rate to answer questions in about 2 s, 5 questions are the limit. These 5 questions should fit on one or two screens on a smartphone at most. At first, we analyzed each parameter and grouped it to *system* and *user* tasks. While the former ones can be performed automatically by the system, user tasks require active user attention. We filtered the final two lists based on relevance derived from the empirical study. Since there are only five parameters remaining, we decided to reduce the threshold value to 0.4 so that we finally have 12 parameters. As received perception of exertion (RPE) is close to the threshold value, we also include it into the final set.

There're five parameters that are requested before workout: psyche, nutrition, sleep, impairment (injury/disease), and alcohol consumption. We decided to summarize disease and injury as one parameter because it's only interesting if there's any physiological impairment before doing sports. After workout, the user is requested for three additional parameters: training partner, injury/disease, and RPE. While the question about training partner is a simple selection between "yes" or "no", injury/disease and RPE are rated via a smiley Likert scale.

In addition to manually entered data, three more parameters are detected automatically. Although training duration has a relevance value less than 0.4 (see Fig. 1), the system will save this information because of the easy tracking possibility. Furthermore, the system can use current location data to request different weather information including wind speed, cloudiness, rain, temperature and humidity. Although only temperature is a relevant parameter according to our empirical study, we also include the remaining weather values because there is no additional effort.

Now that we have our final parameter definition, we need some knowledge as a basis for the rule-based expert system. For this, we created a rule catalogue that consists of over 70 rules based on contributions about internal and external parameters, and findings of our empirical study. Each rule consists of at least one condition and one or more conclusions/actions. They can be read as "IF *condition* THEN *action*". The following Table 2 shows an excerpt of the knowledge base that we use.

Table 2. Some rules of our knowledge base

No.	Condition	Action
R6	ill | pain	2 days training break & resumption 75% of maximum performance
R7	temperature > 28 °C	reduction 75% of maximum performance & reduction training duration 50% & fluid intake 1.0 l/h
R14	temperature > 40 °C	abort workout
R16	heavy solar radiation & windless	light training clothes & sun hat & reduction 75% of maximum performance
R17	humidity > 50%	reduction 75% of maximum performance
R18	rain | hail | snow	rainproof training clothes & warm training clothes & reduction 75% of maximum performance
R19	temperature > 28 °C & humidity > 80% & windless	high heat stroke risk
R20	high heat stroke risk	reduction 50% of maximum performance & training duration < 30 min.
R26	high alcohol consumption	deterioration of sleeping behavior & increasing disease probability & abort workout
R29	on an empty stomach	training duration 50% & reduction of maximum performance up to 30%
R34	trainings partner	positive influence to psyche, RPE, training duration
R36	bad psyche state	reduction training duration
R40	up to 2 h after meal	abort training
R41	training time 4 p.m.–7 p.m.	top condition
R42	top condition	intensive strength training | intensive endurance training | technically demanding sports
R49	after intensive workout	training break 1 day | change type of sport | change muscle group
R63	bad sleep (tired)	decreasing performance & bad psyche | decreasing RPE
R68	sleeping time < 7 h	maximum performance 80% & increasing injury risk

4 Prototype

Our prototype is an Android app especially designed to support TrainOXY™ sensors. After tapping on "Live Mode" in main menu, weather information is gathered automatically on the basis of the user's location. Subsequently, the user is asked to rate the five pre-workout parameters psyche, nutrition, alcohol consumption, sleep, and impairment (see Fig. 2).

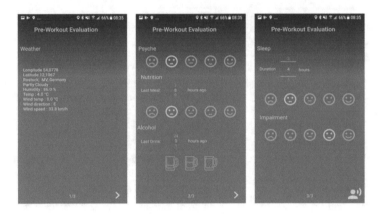

Fig. 2. Pre-workout evaluation

Based on this data our expert system starts processing ("firing") the rules of the knowledge base via forward chaining. This means the inference machine executes every action whose conditions are true. Hereby, new facts can be added to the knowledge base, which in turn can cause more rules to be fired. For instance, if temperature is above 28 °C and humidity is above 80% and it's windless (R19 in Table 2), a new fact is reasoned that there is a high heat stroke risk. This fact will trigger rule R20 that leads to two new facts: reduction to 50% of maximum performance and training duration less than 30 min. The reasoning process is repeated until no more rule is executable. Subsequently, the knowledge base is analyzed and shows the results of the pre-workout analysis in terms of virtual coach advices (left picture in Fig. 3). Here, it's recommend to reduce both training performance and duration. In live mode, this will automatically trigger messages like "Limit: 70%, Reduce Performance!", that appears if one of the user's measured performance parameters is above 70% of maximum value (center picture in Fig. 3). The reference values (e.g. maximum, minimum, average) are values the system has recorded of the last 10% of workouts where the sportsmen had given the corresponding answer in a post-workout test with the same pre-workout-evaluation answers. When no workout with the same answers is found it takes the last workout where the most of the pre-workout-evaluation answers match. If it is the first workout at all, then rules that are based on these values are simply ignored. For example, for the maximum value (subjective limit) of the sportsmen the system searches for workouts with the same answers in the pre-workout evaluation. It takes 10% (fixed value) of the previous matching workouts, but at least 10 (fixed value) so that old workouts do not influence his profile. The average of the maximal values of the workouts of all recorded values will be the new limit. The maximum value of one type of value (e.g. SmO2) workout is the average of the top 10% (fixed value) of all recorded values of the workout.

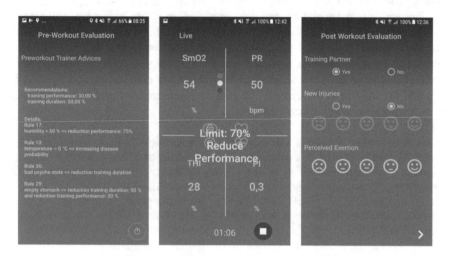

Fig. 3. Virtual coach advices and post-workout evaluation

After finishing a workout, the user presses the stop button that will open the post-workout evaluation form (right picture in Fig. 3). Here, three parameters must be specified: training partner (yes or no), injuries caused by this workout, and overall received perception of exertion (RPE). All information including pre-workout parameters, live mode data (every Bluetooth package of the sensor data in one work and their summary of min/max/average), and post-workout parameters are stored in a database so that the user can review and analyze his sport progress workout for workout. With the visible representation of the workout data as a graph but especially the fired rules in the workout the trainer/the sportsman himself can adapt an external managed training plan.

5   Summary

In this contribution, we described a general method to develop an expert system for dynamically adapting workout sessions of athletes. At first, an extensive literature research was necessary to detect relevant parameters that influence sport performance. Then we took those parameters and conducted an empirical study in order to find out what the most important parameters are. This was necessary to minimize the cognitive load of people using our mobile app by reducing the number of self-assessments users have to do before and after workout sessions. Current prototype in form of an Android application was demonstrated to show the functionality of our approach.

As the next step, we will extend the application for professional sports by adding additional parameters. This will include an energy calculator. Based on detailed nutrition information about macronutrients and micronutrients (e.g. derived from FDDB), and personal data such as height, weight, sex, age, and somatype, daily calorie requirement and consumption can be calculated in order to further optimize the manually created training plans. Furthermore, we will include data-driven machine learning approaches in order to learn new rules based on user statistics. This can be realized as personal rules for each individual and as general rules (in addition to our current knowledge base) that are derived from data of all users. In our last step, we will evaluate our solution by testing the app with a huge number of participants consisting of recreational and professional athletes.

Acknowledgement. We would like to thank TBI Technologie-Beratungs-Institut GmbH for funding University of Rostock's sub-project Train4U. Furthermore, TrainOXY™ is financially supported by the European Union under the European Regional Development Fund (ERDF), Mecklenburg-Western Pomerania's Operational Programme 2014–2020. Special thanks go to our project partners OXY4 GmbH, and Faculty of Engineering, Department Mechanical Engineering/Process and Environmental Engineering, University of Wismar for the work on the cooperative project.

References

Jha, S.N.: Near infrared spectroscopy. In: Nondestructive Evaluation of Food Quality, pp. 141–212. Springer, Heidelberg (2010)

Birrer, R.B., Levine, R.: Performance parameters in children and adolescent athletes. Sports Med. **4**(3), 211–227 (1987)

Dahl, K.D.: External Factors and Athletic Performance. Senior Honors Theses, 347 (2013). https://digitalcommons.liberty.edu/honors/347

Chaouachi, M., Chaouachi, A., Chamari, K., Chtara, M., Feki, Y., Amri, M., Trudeau, F.: Effects of dominant somatotype on aerobic capacity trainability. Br. J. Sports Med. **39**(12), 954–959 (2005)

Phillips, E., Davids, K., Renshaw, I., Portus, M.: Expert performance in sport and the dynamics of talent development. Sports Med. **40**(4), 271–283 (2010)

Ericsson, K.A.: Peak performance and age: an examination of peak performance in sports. In: Successful Aging: Perspectives from the Behavioral Sciences, pp. 164–196 (1990)

McPherson, S.L., Thomas, J.R.: Relation of knowledge and performance in boys' tennis: age and expertise. J. Exp. Child Psychol. **48**(2), 190–211 (1989)

Raglin, J.S.: Psychological factors in sport performance. Sports Med. **31**(12), 875–890 (2001)

Williams, J.M.E.: Applied Sport Psychology: Personal Growth to Peak Performance. Mayfield Publishing Co., Mountain View (1993)

Williams, M.H.: Nutrition for health, fitness and sport, 5th edn. WCB/McGraw-Hill, Boston (1999)

Myer, G.D., Faigenbaum, A.D., Chu, D.A., Falkel, J., Ford, K.R., Best, T.M., Hewett, T.E.: Integrative training for children and adolescents: techniques and practices for reducing sports-related injuries and enhancing athletic performance. Physician Sportsmed. **39**(1), 74–84 (2011)

Savis, J.C.: Sleep and athletic performance: overview and implications for sport psychology. Sports Psychol. **8**(2), 111–125 (1994)

Butt, J., Weinberg, R., Culp, B.: Exploring mental toughness in NCAA athletes. J. Intercoll. Sports **3**(2), 316–332 (2010)

Nippert, A.H., Smith, A.M.: Psychologic stress related to injury and impact on sport performance. Phys. Med. Rehabil. Clin. Am. **19**(2), 399–418 (2008)

Shirreffs, S.M., Maughan, R.J.: The effect of alcohol on athletic performance. Curr. Sports Med. Rep. **5**(4), 192–196 (2006)

Williams, M.H.: Dietary supplements and sports performance: minerals. J. Int. Soc. Sports Nutr. **2**(1), 43 (2005)

Borg, G.A.: Psychophysical bases of perceived exertion. Med. Sci. Sports Exerc. **14**(5), 377–381 (1982)

Vihma, T.: Effects of weather on the performance of marathon runners. Int. J. Biometeorol. **54**(3), 297–306 (2010)

Reilly, T., Atkinson, G., Waterhouse, J.: Chronobiology and physical performance. Exerc. Sports Sci. **24**, 351–372 (2000)

Atkinson, G., Reilly, T.: Circadian variation in sports performance. Sports Med. **21**(4), 292–312 (1996)

Borresen, J., Lambert, M.I.: The quantification of training load, the training response and the effect on performance. Sports Med. **39**(9), 779–795 (2009)

Andersson, H., Ekblom, B., Krustrup, P.: Elite football on artificial turf versus natural grass: movement patterns, technical standards, and player impressions. J. Sports Sci. **26**(2), 113–122 (2008)

Kenney, W.L., Wilmore, J., Costill, D.: Physiology of Sport and Exercise, 6th edn. Human Kinetics, Champaign (2015)

Timmerman, E., De Water, J., Kachel, K., Reid, M., Farrow, D., Savelsbergh, G.: The effect of equipment scaling on children's sport performance: the case for tennis. J. Sports Sci. **33**(10), 1093–1100 (2015)

Thornes, J.E.: The effect of weather on sport. Weather **32**(7), 258–268 (1977)

Siegel, R., Laursen, P.B.: Keeping your cool. Sports Med. **42**(2), 89–98 (2012)

Lindberg, A.S., Malm, C., Hammarström, D., Oksa, J., Tonkonogi, M.: Maximal work capacity and performance depends warm-up procedure and environmental but not inspired air temperatures. J. Exerc. Physiol. Online **15**(1), 26–39 (2012)

Komarow, H.D., Postolache, T.T.: Seasonal allergy and seasonal decrements in athletic performance. Clin. Sports Med. **24**(2), e35–e50 (2005)

Huang, K.Y.: Challenges in human-computer interaction design for mobile devices. In: Proceedings of the World Congress on Engineering and Computer Science, vol. 1, pp. 236–241 (2009)

From Sensor Data to Coaching in Alpine Skiing – A Software Design to Facilitate Immediate Feedback in Sports

Richard Brunauer[1]([✉]), Wolfgang Kremser[1], and Thomas Stöggl[2]

[1] Salzburg Research Forschungsgesellschaft GmbH, Jakob-Haringer-Straße 5,
5020 Salzburg, Austria
{richard.brunauer,wolfgang.
kremser}@salzburgresearch.at
[2] Department of Sport and Exercise Science, University of Salzburg,
Schlossallee 49, 5400 Hallein, Austria
thomas.stoeggl@sbg.ac.at

Abstract. Thanks to wearable sensor technologies, it has become feasible to quantify human kinematics cheaply and comprehensively during sports. However, it is often left to the user to infer any qualitative information from the data, leaving them confused about their performance and what actions to take next. This paper presents a high-level process to transform sensor data into immediate expert feedback in the form of coaching instructions. Individual aspects of process and software design are discussed based on an example implementation for Alpine skiing. In detail, this paper aims to (1) describe the transformation from raw sensor data into coaching instructions from a software engineering and data-centric perspective; (2) propose a high-level software design for coaching applications in sports that facilitates historical as well as immediate data analytics; (3) decompose the task of developing coaching applications into independent, manageable research subtasks; and (4) show software engineers which data structures and interactions to implement.

Keywords: Alpine skiing · Real-time coaching · Software design · Sensor data

1 Introduction

The smartphone has long been identified as a promising gateway to publicly promote physical activity. Today's app marketplaces offer a vast number of fitness apps, both free and paid [1]. Coupled with the overall miniaturization of sensing hardware, it is now possible to gather and display a wide array of information about activity and motion. However, ordinary users of such systems lack the expert knowledge required to leverage these data [2]. To truly create value for these users, developers have to provide coaching that is based on expert knowledge and scientific evaluation. This is reflected in the number of app downloads [1].

That being said, getting such an application off the ground is no small task. How do you get from raw sensor readings to immediate and relevant coaching instructions? This paper is the result of an interdisciplinary research effort between sports scientists,

© Springer Nature Switzerland AG 2020
M. Lames et al. (Eds.): IACSS 2019, AISC 1028, pp. 86–95, 2020.
https://doi.org/10.1007/978-3-030-35048-2_11

data scientists and software engineers to create a coaching application for Alpine skiing. First it introduces a general model of coaching applications that aims to outline the steps necessary to transform raw sensor data into coaching instructions. It goes on to discuss this model from both a data-centric and a software engineering perspective. After presenting the resulting implementation which builds on reactive programming, the paper discusses the software design's role in supporting the interdisciplinary development process.

2   A Prototypic Coaching Application: Alpine Skiing

Providing coaching instructions in Alpine skiing is a common task for ski instructors. They look at the performance of their students and give personalized instructions based on their own knowledge and experience (e.g. how to correct a "sloppy" turn). Beyond that, it is mandatory to ensure that the student skis safely relative to their skiing abilities. Digital aids are limited in terms hardware, software and data analytics (e.g. size limitations, energy efficiency, and computational performance). All of this makes digitizing coaching instruction difficult.

Recognizing techniques is a general prerequisite for a wider, more useful set of application scenarios in sports, including coaching. This is comparable to activity recognition in the field of wearable computing. In a common activity recognition process, the user gets equipped with one or multiple sensors near their body. These sensors capture physical phenomena (e.g. acceleration, rotational velocity) over a certain amount of time. After data generation, the resulting multivariate time series is processed to recognize activities, such as sitting, walking or exercising.

The *Activity Recognition Chain* (ARC) [3] is a standard process to derive activity information from a multivariate time series. It divides the whole classification task into four steps (Fig. 1).

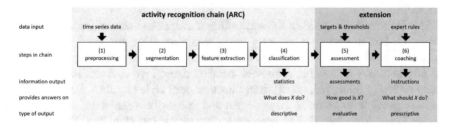

Fig. 1. The extended ARC extends the ARC by adding steps for assessing and coaching.

The ARC standard can be adapted to sports by defining "activity" as "using a certain technique within a discipline". Additionally, we propose an extension of the ARC by adding the steps of assessing and coaching. This extended ARC conceptualizes how data are transformed into coaching instructions and how coaching systems can look like on a high level.

How can the concept of the extended ARC be applied to Alpine skiing? To gather data, ski equipment like skis or ski boots can be retrofitted with digital sensors. Popular sensors in sports are inertial measurement units (IMUs; acceleration, angular velocity, magnetic field strength) and global navigation satellite systems (GNSS; position data). Additional sensors could measure temperature, air pressure or sole pressure. The collected data are either stored locally on devices or are transmitted wirelessly (Bluetooth, WiFi) to a processing unit (e.g. smartphone). Scientific approaches and recent consumer devices following this approach are [4, 5] and Snowcookie, Carv or PIQ Robot. For this paper, we adopt the setup proposed by Martinez et al. [6], where wireless IMUs were situated on the posterior upper cuff of each ski boot. The measurements were recorded with 64 Hz, synchronized, and provided as a single equidistant and multivariate time series.

Martinez et al. [6] presented two processing steps. First, data were filtered (lowpass Butterworth with 0.5 Hz) and processed with simple mathematical methods. This corresponds with the ARC's preprocessing step (step 1, cf. Fig. 1). The resulting, relatively smooth signal showed turn switch points as local extrema of the angular velocity on the roll axis. Identifying these local extrema, i.e. cutting the signal into turns, represents ARC's segmentation step (step 2, cf. Fig. 1). Based on such a turn detection algorithm we continue to discuss how further processing for obtaining coaching instructions might look like.

The ARC's next step after segmentation is feature extraction (step 3, cf. Fig. 1). By learning where turn switches, and therefore turns, happen it becomes possible to derive additional information for each turn. For example: (1) turn duration, turn direction, speed, radius, distance; (2) acceleration on roll axis, centrifugal forces; (3) edge angle, symmetry between left and right edge angle; (4) detailed reconstruction of motion trajectory during a turn; (5) pressure distribution of dynamic pressure profile (if pressure sensors are available); (6) vertical speed, difference in altitude, piste's inclination rating (7) turn phases etc. All in all, knowing the start and end timestamps of a turn, together with the preprocessed signals allows for deriving a lot of turn specific information.

This information is used in the succeeding classification step of the ARC (step 4, cf. Fig. 1). For example, maximum g-force, maximum edge angle, edge angle symmetry and speed of a turn are plausible candidates to recognize carving turns. At the end of this step it is possible to provide detailed descriptive statistics that consider a piste's difficulty (blue, red, black), turn direction, turn style or radius. For example, it becomes possible to compare edge angles and speeds between short, mid and long carving turns. After step 4 it is possible to answer the question (Fig. 1): What does X do?

The idea of our extension of the ARC's is to answer (Fig. 1): How *good* is X? For the assessment step (step 5, cf. Fig. 1), let us assume that we have several advanced, expert and/or world cup skiers. All of them go through the exact same analytics procedure, producing a number of comparable features. It is then possible for sports scientists to derive or postulate targets for students to work towards. These targets are modeled with threshold values or a (subjective) scoring system. By comparing turn features of the student with targets', each turn gets one or more assessments These assessments can either be presented to the student directly (e.g. via a smartphone app) or can be forwarded to the coaching step (step 6, cf. Fig. 1). The rules for deciding which coaching instruction would be proper can be digitized (e.g. decision trees) and stored. For instance, an app could play a proper audio cue whenever the student triggers one of the coaching rules by having bad pressure distribution.

However, the previous described process is challenging from several perspectives: (1) a reliable and non-obstructive hardware with a sufficient power supply is needed; (2) the data analytics and the algorithm design are not trivial. Requiring immediate feedback disqualifies a lot of mathematical approaches (e.g. zero-lag Butterworth filter); (3) a scientific evaluation of all components, algorithms and models is methodically challenging and requires much effort from sport scientists; (4) deployment of the final analytics process is complex. And finally, (5) a software architecture that integrates all of the above. Challenge (1) concerns hardware issues. Challenge (2), (3) and (4) depend on the sport in question. Nevertheless, it is possible to identify a software architecture that provides a general solution for challenge (5).

3 The Data-Centric Perspective

The extended ARC divides the data analytics process into major "semantic" steps. In this section we focus on the data structures passed between these steps. Figure 2 shows this data-centric perspective. The input of the process are sensor data from different sources which we assume have been synchronized and resampled with missing data imputated. Hence, the input is an equidistant, more or less complete multivariate time series. The output of the process are descriptive statistics, quality assessments and coaching instructions.

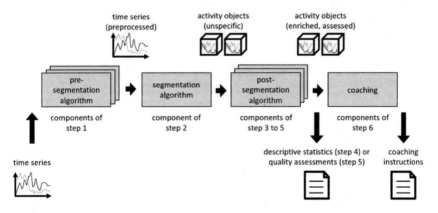

Fig. 2. The data-centric perspective on the extended ARC.

In step 1, raw signals are processed to create the prerequisites for later steps. Such a step usually contains GNSS data processing (spatio-temporal algorithms), filtering (low-pass filter, Kalman filter), smoothing, fusion of IMU data, conversations of units or calibration of sensor data. The result of this step is again a multivariate time series with substituted or added signals (i.e. columns).

The segmentation in step 2 is the most important step when talking about data structures. It cuts the multivariate time series signals into segments. This segmentation should not be done arbitrarily. Rather, cuts should represent the start and end timestamps of clearly distinct reoccurring or cyclic activities of the specific sport. Examples for such reoccurring or cyclic activities are turns in Alpine skiing, strokes in tennis, steps during running or even shots in golf. These activities are the smallest unit of interests and the basis for deriving coaching instructions. In terms of data structure, the time series segments are wrapped and passed on to the next step as an *activity object*, e.g. a turn object.

For the rest of the process there is no necessity to change the data structure of the activity object. Step 3, the feature extraction, only adds information derived from already present data. These derived data are additional metadata (as member variables) or additional time series data (cf. Fig. 3). The derived information is used in the succeeding assessment and classification steps. Sometimes it can be necessary to normalize the time series signals. Such a normalization would be part of step 3. In Alpine skiing for instance, turns can have durations between 0.5 and 5 s. To compare turns, it is common to normalize (i.e. resample) all turns to a fictive duration from 0 to 100%.

Step 4, the classification, assigns a technique to the activity object. For example, in Alpine skiing turns might be assigned to the classes *snow plow*, *carving* or *skidded turns*. Additionally, it would be possible to present at least some descriptive statistics after step 4 or quality assessments after step 5. To do that, the set of activity objects are aggregated using aggregation criteria, e.g. aggregate all carving turns with long radius on blue pistes. All information necessary for aggregation exists in each activity object as metadata. Thus, the aim of preprocessing, segmentation, feature extraction and classification is to enrich the activity objects with all information needed for aggregation and assessment. Finally, at step 6, activity objects are mapped to coaching instructions.

Turn #7	metadata (statistics)		time series (normalized)				step 3
	key value pairs		time	acc X	gyro X	GPS	...
step 2	duration	3.43 seconds	0 %	0.51	5.21	lat,lon	
	direction	left	1 %	0.52	5.18	lat,lon	
	distance	51.5 m	2 %	0.59	4.59	lat,lon	
	radius	18 m	...				
step 3	incline	blue	metadata (assessment)				step 5
	balance	-0.8 (outside)	key value pairs				
	speed	15.0 m/s	carving score	5			
step 4	turn style	carving	max speed	18.1 m/s			
	...	...	...	...			

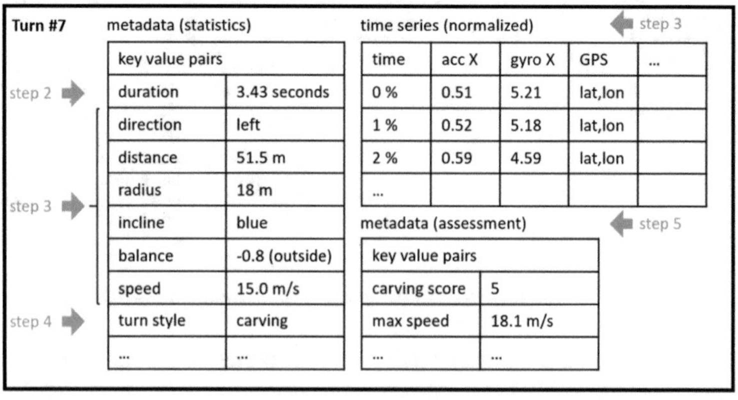

Fig. 3. Activity object *Turn*: Filled with some exemplary values for Alpine skiing.

4   The Software Engineering Perspective

In order to provide timely feedback it is crucial that a digital coaching system immediately processes incoming data. This poses unique challenges regarding software design:

1. *Data is unbounded* – From the system's viewpoint, it is not possible to predict when the dataset is going to be complete. The system must expect incoming data at any time. Consequently, it is also not possible to anticipate the size of the complete data.
2. *Data arrives small* – Instead of large bulks, data arrives in small units, or even as a single data point. This means that the ingestion rate, i.e. the rate at which the processing system has to handle new data, can be very high. The ingestion rate largely depends on the sampling rate of the data producers.
3. *The data is out of order* – Due to the nature of wireless data transmission and concurrency, data packages might be received in a quasi-random order. Therefore, the data's time of arrival is unfit to establish a before-after relationship between data points.
4. *The data itself is not of interest* – At any point during the extended ARC process, some of the collected data could be discarded because they do not provide any more information. Note though that the whole dataset might still be useful during software and algorithm development, as it allows debugging and experimentation without having to record data.

Cugola and Margara [7] would place an application with these requirements into what they call the *Information Flow Processing* (IFP) domain: Data are generated by multiple distributed and heterogeneous sources (e.g. different IMUs) and continuously "flow" to the center of the system, called IFP engine, for processing. This requires no explicit user action; processing starts or continues as soon as there is new data available. Once the IFP engine calculated the results, it is no longer necessary to keep the original data (except for debugging). Finally, the results are forwarded to a sink where the information is somehow used (e.g. visualized on dashboard).

It would be possible to view the whole of the extended ARC as a single IFP engine. However, this monolithic design is highly inflexible and creates strong dependencies. If data or sports scientists want to add, modify or exchange individual parts (i.e. sub-algorithms like g-force or edge angle calculation) of the extended ARC they have to rely on the software engineer to implement their ideas. This stifles fast iteration cycles and fosters software complicity and dependencies. This is problematic especially when project goals are shifting due to new emerging requirements and gained scientific insight.

Instead, we propose to model the extended ARC as a series of one or more independent IFP engines. As proposed in Sect. 3, each IFP engine completes a clearly defined sub-task and forwards its result to the next IFP engine. Effectively, each IFP engine acts as both a source and sink. We will call such a chain of IFP engines an IFP pipeline, illustrated in Fig. 4. In this setting, the exemplary g-force and edge angle sub-algorithms can be independently researched, designed and implemented. Thus, they can be treated as independent IFP engines. However, the order of execution remains important. Some IFP engines may expect derived data from previous steps to already be present (Fig. 2).

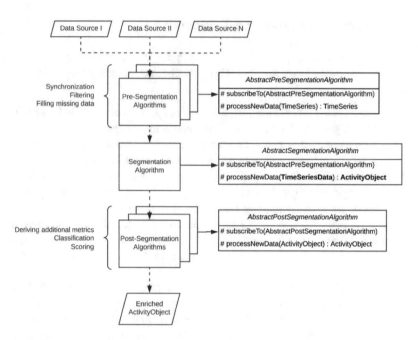

Fig. 4. Illustration of an IFP pipeline that implements the extended ARC. Dashed arrows illustrate the flow of data. The transition from time series data to an activity object in bold.

To implement the IFP pipeline, one needs components that are able to react to newly available data in an asynchronous manner. The *Observer Pattern* [8] is a well-known design pattern in software engineering fit for implementing such components. A component called *Observer* subscribes to another component called *Observable*. Every time the Observable has new data available, it notifies its observers and forwards the data.

Although the general idea is simple, embedding it in a multi-threaded, asynchronous setting is far more complex. The library *ReactiveX* [9] abstracts these issues away and provides additional operators for manipulating sequences of data. ReactiveX is available for the majority of popular programming languages. The Alpine skiing pipeline was implemented in Java (with RxJava). In her book chapter "ReactiveX and RxJava", Maglie [10] provides a further introduction with code examples. Henceforth the terms "Observer" and "Observable" refer to their specific implementation in ReactiveX.

Finally, we can describe the whole implementation layout. The extended ARC (≙IFP pipeline, cf. Fig. 1) consists of a series of connected highly independent processing steps (≙IFP engines). Each processing step acts as both an Observable (≙data source) and an Observer (≙data sink). At some point in the pipeline (≙step 2 in the extended ARC) the time series signal is segmented into activity objects (cf. Fig. 2). The implementation therefore distinguishes between processing steps before and after this segmentation, as well as the segmentation step itself.

5   Implementation and Results

The extended ARC was implemented according to Sect. 4 using RxJava. Its individual components, i.e. algorithms, were developed according to Martinez et al. [6] in order to detect Alpine skiing turns within IMU signals. Additional algorithms have been added over time. The following Java code snippet illustrates the instantiation, configuration, and starting of such a pipeline:

```
AlgorithmPipeline.Factory factory = new AlgorithmPipeline.Factory()
        .addAlgorithm(PreprocessingAlgorithm.class)  // pre, step 1
        .addAlgorithm(TurnDetection.class)           // seg., step 2
        .addAlgorithm(EdgingAlgorithm.class)         // post, step 3
        .addAlgorithm(GForceAlgorithm.class)         // post, step 3
        .addAlgorithm(TurnClassifier.class)          // post, step 4
        .addAlgorithm(ScoringAlgorithm.class);       // post, step 5

//Signal source is the source of the IMU data
AlgorithmPipeline pipeline = pipelineFactory.build(signalSource);
pipeline.start();
```

The resulting application supports two modes of operation: live and historic. In live mode, the pipeline runs on a smartphone that is directly connected to the two IMUs via Bluetooth. When an activity object, i.e. a turn, is detected, it is segmented, enriched, and output immediately.

The pipeline's second mode of operation, historic, takes a CSV file containing pre-recorded IMU data as input and then emulates the behavior of live data. The result is a CSV file containing the enriched turns that were detected within the input file. Furthermore, each component writes its intermediate results into its respective CSV file.

While it was originally planned to deploy the pipeline on Android smartphones, the need for an iOS port of the application emerged eventually. The port uses RxSwift which is ReactiveX's implementation for the Swift programming language.

6   Discussion

This paper presents a software design that aims to facilitate the transformation from raw sensor data to relevant and immediate coaching instructions. It is part of the scientific output from two application-oriented projects between 2015 and 2019. The development team for these projects was a cooperation between a team of sports scientists, and a second team consisting of data scientists and software engineers.

The interdisciplinary nature of the development team has shown to be very constructive. Each expert group complemented the skills of the others: Sports scientists know how to plan and execute the studies required for data collection, both in the laboratory and the field. With their domain knowledge they are able to interpret the kinesiological phenomena that occur in a given sport. They might also have access to specialized equipment with which to measure metrics of interest. However, they might lack in experience and knowledge about data analytics methods that go beyond statistics. Data scientists can fill this gap. They are familiar with modern data analytics tools and methods, and are skilled in translating application requirements into data requirements. Together, sports and data scientists enable each other to create algorithms based on a clean data generation process, domain knowledge, and the optimal data analytics methods. Lastly, software engineers build the data infrastructure and provide appropriate interfaces to abstract away concerns not directly related to algorithm development, like concurrency control or data structures. This enables sports and data scientists to quickly test their hypotheses and in turn speeds up algorithm development.

Nonetheless, this collaboration posed challenges as well. One of them was organizing and assigning the individual research topics. Introducing the extended ARC and basing the processing pipeline on this rather general concept was helpful in establishing broad categories and a common vocabulary. By defining expected input and output at each step of the extended ARC, it served as a point of orientation during the development of individual components.

Another issue was the inclusion of individual results into the growing pipeline. Several master and PhD students were involved who worked on single topics (e.g. g-force, edge angle calculation). How should their findings be integrated? The pipeline design made adding or replacing components easy. However, it did not provide interfaces for popular scripting languages like R, Python or Matlab. Since most of the algorithm code was provided in one of these languages, translating them into Java was a necessary step done manually by the data science team. This also meant that the sport science team could not interact directly with the pipeline. Instead, they locally processed the intermediate CSV output created by the pipeline components outside of the pipeline itself. This process was not ideal, it made the sport science team dependent on the data science team. As scripting languages grow in popularity, especially in fields that rely on statistics, it becomes necessary to provide appropriate interfaces.

The second goal of the software design was the provision of immediate coaching instructions. What is considered immediate depends on the underlying feedback model. For example, in some feedback models it is necessary to give feedback only seconds after a turn, while in others it is sufficient to provide coaching after the skiing day. The pipeline itself does not impose any restrictions on how fast data can be processed, but the design of the components does.

Some mathematical operations, like a zero-lag Butterworth filter, become infeasible because they produce different numerical results in live and historic mode. A moving average does not work properly if the data available is smaller than the window size. Nonetheless, the results from the pipeline should be numerically equal between streaming and historical mode. Thus, some of the mathematical functions have to buffer data before producing results, which delays further processing and consequently delays the feedback.

Finally, the translation from RxJava to RxSwift was relatively easy due to the ReactiveX framework not being language specific. Although the syntax might change, the concept and its components' semantics and names stay the same. Overall, ReactiveX was a good choice as a framework for implementing the pipeline design.

7 Conclusion

The proposed high-level software design structures the task of immediate coaching feedback as follows: (1) The extended Activity Recognition Chain decomposes the whole task into a group of six general semantic steps. (2) From a data-centric perspective, it is sufficient to provide only two data structures, one for time series (sensor signals) and one for activity objects (turn objects). (3) The concepts of Information Flow Processing (IFP), Observer Pattern and Reactive Programming allow decomposition of the coaching tasks into highly independent components aligned in a loosely coupled processing pipeline. Components can be treated separately in research, algorithm design and algorithm implementation. They are easy to add, change, exchange and debug.

Acknowledgements. This work was partly funded by the Austrian Federal Ministry for Transport, Innovation and Technology, the Austrian Federal Ministry for Digital and Economic Affairs, and the federal state of Salzburg.

References

1. Bondaronek, P., Alkhaldi, G., Slee, A., Hamilton, F.L., Murray, E.: Quality of publicly available physical activity apps: Review and content analysis. JMIR mHealth uHealth **6**(3), e53 (2018)
2. Kranz, M., Möller, A., Hammerla, N., Diewald, S.: The mobile fitness coach: towards individualized skill assessment using personalized mobile devices. Pervasive Mob. Comput. **9**(2), 203–215 (2012)
3. Roggen, D., Magnenat, S., Waibel, M., Troester, G.: Wearable computing - designing and sharing activity-recognition systems across platforms. IEEE Robot. Autom. Mag **18**(2) (2011)
4. Yu, G., Jang, Y.J., Kim, J., Kim, J.H., Kim, H.Y., Kim, K., Panday, S.B.: Potential of IMU sensors in performance analysis of professional alpine skiers. Sensors **16**(4), 463 (2016)
5. Fasel, B., Spörri, J., Schütz, P., Lorenzetti, S., Aminian, K.: An inertial sensor-based method for estimating the athlete's relative joint center positions and center of mass kinematics in alpine ski racing. Front. Physiol. **8**, 850 (2017)
6. Martinez, A., Jahnel, R., Buchecker, M., Snyder, C., Brunauer, R., Stöggl, T.: Development of an automatic alpine skiing turn detection algorithm based on a simple sensor setup. Sensors **19**(4), 902 (2019)
7. Cugola, G., Margara, A.: Processing flows of information: From data stream to complex event processing. J. ACM Comput. Surv. **44**(3), 1–62 (2012)
8. Gamma, E.: Design Patterns: Elements of Reusable Object-Oriented Software. Pearson Education (1995)
9. ReactiveX. http://reactivex.io. Accessed 22 Mar 2019
10. Maglie, A.: ReactiveX and RxJava. In: Reactive Java Programming, Apress (2016)

Biomechanical Analysis of Technique of Highly Skilled Weightlifters with the Application of Mathematical Modeling and High-Speed Video Recording

Leonid A. Khasin[✉]

Research Institute of Information Technologies of Moscow State Academy
of Physical Education, Malakhovka, Moscow Region, Russia
niit@mgafk.ru

Abstract. The biomechanical characteristics of the technique of highly skilled weightlifters are described. The method of motion detection was high-speed video, mathematical modeling and filtering algorithms were used as methods of analysis. Differences in the microstructure of movement in successful and unsuccessful attempts are revealed. The spatio-temporal, kinematic and dynamic characteristics of the snatch are determined. The method of calculation of vertical and horizontal forces applied by a weightlifter to the bar is described.

Keywords: Technique of snatch · Biomechanical analysis · Technique of highly skilled weightlifters · Mathematical modeling of human motion · High-speed video recording · Microstructure of weightlifting exercises

1 Introduction

The Research Institute of Information Technologies of the Moscow State Academy of Physical Education has been carrying research of the technique of highly skilled athletes for years, using high-speed video recording, mathematical modeling and modern methods of data analysis. We have obtained new results that go beyond the framework of previous ideas, and often contradict them. This can be explained both by the evolution of the technique of highly skilled athletes and by improving the means of recording and analyzing human movements.

The considerable number of works is devoted to various aspects of the analysis of the equipment of weight-lifters of high qualification ([1–4], etc.). Space-time, kinetic, dynamic characteristics of snatch were studied. However, the following aspects were studied poorly: (a) vertical and horizontal forces of interaction of the athlete with a barbell; (b) a role of a repulse of a bar when performing snatch; (c) biomechanical characteristics during a repulse; (d) microstructure of snatch of a bar, identification of differences in biomechanical characteristics of successful and unsuccessful attempts, etc.

We present the methods for the analysis of the technique of weight-lifters of high qualification. These methods were developed on the basis of our previous research.

M. Lames et al. (Eds.): IACSS 2019, AISC 1028, pp. 96–105, 2020.
https://doi.org/10.1007/978-3-030-35048-2_12

In the process of the research the following problems were solved: (1) determination of space-time, kinetic, dynamic characteristics of snatch; (2) development of a method of calculation of vertical and horizontal forces of interaction of the athlete with a barbell; (3) development of a method of calculation of biomechanical characteristics of interaction of the athlete with a barbell; (4) definition of a microstructure of a snatch of a bar, identification of differences in biomechanical characteristics of successful and unsuccessful attempts.

We studied space-time, kinetic and dynamic characteristics of snatch. The comparative analysis of successful and unsuccessful approaches was carried out. Research methods include mathematical modeling, the algorithms of filtration and other mathematical methods of the analysis of data developed by us. For registration of the movement high-speed video recording with 250–500 frames per second was used. The analysis of results of high-speed video recording allowed us to develop new phase structure of snatch and to describe the modern equipment of athletes of high qualification. We analyzed more than 120 video records of competitive approaches of world-class athletes, including national team of Russia.

2 Analysis of Spatio-Temporal, Kinematic and Dynamic Characteristics of the Barbell Snatch

The analysis was based on the results of high-speed video recording (250 frames per second) of a snatch performed by a member of the Russian national weightlifting team. The weight of the barbell was 170 kg.

We use the following spatio-temporal characteristics: vertical and horizontal movements of the end of the barbell when performing a snatch (Fig. 1), the time between the end of the final acceleration phase and the beginning of the unsupported phase, the time of the unsupported phase, the maximum height of the barbell liftoff, the height of the bar at the time of landing of the athlete after the unsupported phase [5]. Significant differences in successful and unsuccessful attempts for the last four characteristics were found. The points in Figs. 1, 2 and 3 mark the beginning and end of the interaction of the athlete with the hips ("repulse").

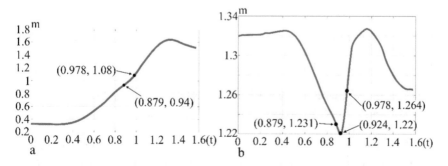

Fig. 1. Vertical (a) and horizontal (b) movement of the end of the barbell

Kinematic characteristics are vertical and horizontal speeds of the end of the barbell when performing a snatch (Fig. 2). Dynamic characteristics are vertical and horizontal acceleration of the barbell end (Fig. 3), as well as vertical and horizontal forces applied by the athlete to the bar [5, 6]. The method of force calculation will be discussed below.

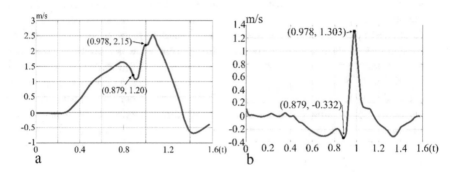

Fig. 2. Vertical (a) and horizontal (b) velocity of the barbell end

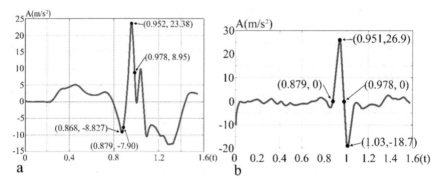

Fig. 3. Vertical (a) and horizontal (b) acceleration of the barbell end

The graphs of horizontal and vertical movements, velocities and accelerations presented above will be used to calculate the horizontal and vertical forces. The greatest interest is the phase of "repulse" of the barbell, at which the maximum acceleration of the barbell end is achieved (Fig. 3).

3 Analysis of Successful and Unsuccessful Attempts in the Snatches of Highly Skilled Weightlifters

The comparative analysis of a microstructure of snatch in successful and unsuccessful attempts of the athlete in the same competitions was carried out. We considered only attempts in which bar weight did not differ or differed no more than on 3 kg. Attempts of 38 athletes, members of national team of Russia on weightlifting, are analyzed.

Significant differences found for the following characteristics: the maximum height of the barbell liftoff (p < 0.00001) and the height of the barbell at the time of landing after the unsupported phase (p < 0.00001), the time of the unsupported phase (p < 0.0001) and the time between the end of the final acceleration phase and the beginning of the unsupported phase (p < 0.01). The average duration of unsupported phases in successful attempts is 0.015 s longer than in unsuccessful ones. The height of the barbell at the time of landing and the maximum height of the barbell in successful attempts is on average 0,015 m higher than in unsuccessful ones [7].

Thus, the maximum height of barbell lifting in the squatting position in a successful attempt was 1144.3 mm, in a failed one – 1125.7 mm (Fig. 4).

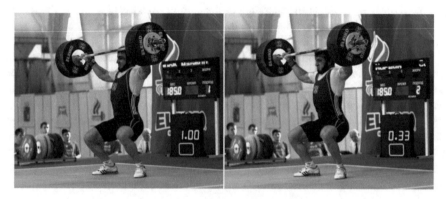

Fig. 4. Posture at the moment of reaching the maximum height of the barbell in the squatting position. Unsuccessful (left) and successful (right) attempts.

As can be seen from Fig. 4, there are characteristic differences in the athlete's posture in the successful and unsuccessful attempts. At the time of reaching the maximum height of the barbell liftoff in the successful attempt, the posture of the athlete is closer to the position of fixing the apparatus: the angles in the ankle, knee and hip joints are smaller than the angles at the time of maximum liftoff height in the failed attempt.

4   Phase Structure of the Snatch

The phase structure of the snatch, which, in addition to traditional phases, includes additional phases and microphases with a duration not exceeding 0.02–0.03 s, was described. These are switching phases, the duration of which is equal to the time from the end of the extension to the beginning of the flexion of the joint and vice versa, for example, the end of the pre-acceleration – the beginning of the amortization phase and the end of the amortization phase – the beginning of the final acceleration phase.

The phase structure also includes a description of such elements of movement as early stepping on toes within the phase of amortization, extension of the hip joint and tilting the shoulders back in the process of performing the phase of amortization and at the beginning of the final acceleration phase, which provides a powerful repulse of the barbell and the creation of significant horizontal and vertical forces. Currently, these elements are, in part or in whole, inherent in the technique of the best athletes. At the same time, according to the recommendations of experts of the past, such performance of the exercises was considered erroneous [5].

5   Method of Calculation of the Vertical Forces Applied by the Athlete to the Bar

To calculate the vertical forces, frontal shooting was performed. The motion was analyzed from the moment of separation of the barbell from the platform to the fixation of the apparatus in the squatting position.

Two methods of calculation of vertical forces were used.

First Method. To calculate the forces applied by the athlete to the barbell, the position of the centers of mass of the weight plate packages and their accelerations were determined. The coordinates of the marked couple of points were used for this purpose. The first point of the couple is the barbell end; the second one is a point on the inner edge of the weight plate stopper. The position of the center of mass of the weight plates was determined for geometric reasons. The coordinates of the marked points allowed determining the coordinates and accelerations of the centers of mass of the weight plates, which were calculated using a digital filter. To find the total force applied by the athlete to the barbell, the following equation was solved:

$$m\bar{a} = \bar{P} - m\bar{g} \tag{1}$$

where m is the mass of the barbell, a is the acceleration of the center of the weight plate package, P is the force applied by the athlete to the barbell, g is acceleration of gravity.

Equation (1) holds for the following assumptions. We consider the vertical movement of the barbell. The initial position is horizontal. During the exercise, the line connecting the ends of the barbell moves in parallel to the starting position. The points of application of forces P are symmetrical with respect to the center of the barbell, the right and left ends of the barbell have identical movement curves. The forces are directed vertically.

The second method uses mathematical modeling, which is based on the equation of the elastic line [8]. To calculate the dynamic characteristics of the barbell movement, a mathematical model was developed, in which the barbell is considered as a steel beam with a constant circular cross section lying on two movable supports moving with acceleration a. The geometric model is shown in Fig. 5. We assume that the weight of the barbell is concentrated at points C and D, and the bar is considered as weightless.

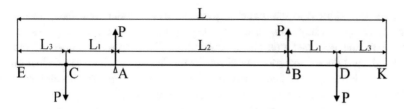

Fig. 5. Design scheme of bending of a steel beam on two supports

Points A and B correspond to the position of the supports (points on the shoulders), points C and D correspond to the centers of mass of weight plate packages, points E and K are marked by the barbell ends.

The deflection of the beam at the points of application of forces C and D can be calculated by formula (2)

$$y_C = y_D - \frac{PL_1^2}{EI}\left(\tfrac{1}{3}L_1 + \tfrac{1}{2}L_2\right) = -P * k_1,$$

where $k_1 = \frac{L_1^2}{EI}\left(\tfrac{1}{3}L_1 + \tfrac{1}{2}L_2\right), E = 2.1 * 10^{11} \text{N/m}^2$ - modulus of elasticity for steel.

(2)

The deflection of the beam at the ends (points E and K) can be calculated by formula (3):

$$y_E = y_C - \frac{PL_1}{EI}\left(\tfrac{1}{2}L_1 + \tfrac{1}{2}L_2\right) * L_3 = y_C - P * k_2 = y_C * \frac{k_1 + k_2}{k_1}, \text{where}$$
$$k_2 = \frac{L_1}{EI}\left(\tfrac{1}{2}L_1 + \tfrac{1}{2}L_2\right) * L_3.$$

(3)

I is the section modulus for a circle of radius R, calculated by formula 4:

$$I = \frac{\pi R_4}{4}.$$

(4)

Using formulas (1), (2) and having the known coordinates of the barbell ends and points of support (the athlete's hands), it is possible to calculate force P at the points of application of forces through the measured deflection value. Using formula (2), it is possible to find force P at points C and D, and knowing the barbell mass – the acceleration at these points.

The accelerations of the barbell end and of the center of weight plate package were obtained.

The calculated values of accelerations of the weight plate packages obtained from the presented model at every moment of the exercise performance were lower than the accelerations of the barbell end. The maximum distinctions of accelerations are reached in the course of a repulse at the same time. The maximum vertical acceleration for the end of a signature stamp is 23.38 m/c², Fig. 3(a). The maximum vertical acceleration of the center of a package of bar pancakes calculated on model was 13.42 m/c².

The forces applied to the barbell calculated on the "filter" and using the model of the beam deflection have similar curves. The amplitudes of the force peaks calculated by each of the two methods are synchronous. The amplitude values of the forces calculated by different methods are close for the moments where the deflection of the bar reaches large values. The maximum force of interaction of the athlete with the barbell, under the assumption that the barbell is a rigid body (Formula (1)), is 564 kgF. In the case where the elastic properties of the bar are taken into account, the maximum vertical force is 394,8 kgF.

6   Calculation of the Horizontal Forces

The method of calculation of the horizontal forces is described in detail in [6]. Shooting was performed from the end side of the bar. To calculate the horizontal forces applied by the athlete to the barbell when performing a snatch, we used curves of movement, speed and acceleration of the barbell end (Figs. 1, 2 and 3). The analysis of the video records and the corresponding processing of the obtained velocity and acceleration curves showed that at the time of "repulse" of the barbell (Fig. 6) there are high horizontal and vertical accelerations of the barbell end and, respectively, high values of the forces.

We considered two cases: the first one is the "repulse" of the barbell by the hips (Fig. 5), in which there are large (400 kgF) instantaneous forces of the athlete's interaction with the barbell. The second one is the horizontal acceleration that occurs when the shoulders are moved. The second acceleration is much lower than the acceleration during the repulse, so, when calculating the horizontal acceleration at times that do not include the "repulse", we consider the barbell as a rigid body.

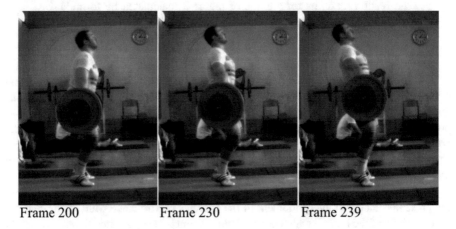

Frame 200   Frame 230   Frame 239

Fig. 6. Process of the barbell "repulse" by the hips

To calculate the forces of the interaction between the athlete and the barbell, we use the bending scheme of the steel beam on two supports at points A and B with a weight in the form of a point mass m at points C and D and with a constant circular cross section (Fig. 4).

The deflection of the beam relative to the supports (athlete's hips) A and B at the points of application of forces C and D can be calculated by formula (2). The deflection of the beam at the ends (point E) is calculated by formula (3):

From Eq. (3), when supports A and B are immovable, one derives the rigid relation between the velocities and accelerations of the bar end and the weight, namely

$$\dot{y}_E = \dot{y}_C \cdot \frac{k_1 + k_2}{k_1}, \ddot{y}_E = \ddot{y}_C \cdot \frac{k_1 + k_2}{k_1}.$$

However, if the supports are movable, the relation between the velocities and accelerations of the bar end and the weight become more complex:

$$\dot{y}_C = \frac{k_2}{k_1 + k_2} \cdot \dot{y}_A + \frac{k_1}{k_1 + k_2} \cdot \dot{y}_E, \ddot{y}_C = \frac{k_2}{k_1 + k_2} \cdot \ddot{y}_A + \frac{k_1}{k_1 + k_2} \cdot \ddot{y}_E. \qquad (5)$$

Thus, with movable supports, the knowledge of the velocity and acceleration of point E alone is not enough to calculate the velocity and acceleration of point C: it is also needed to know the velocity and acceleration of point A.

The beginning and the end of the interaction of the bar with the hips occur at times when the acceleration of the bar end is zero. At these moments, the bar is in a straightened condition, that is, the fulcrum point, the center of mass of the weight and the bar end lie on a straight line. Let S be the displacements of the supports and the bar end during the interaction, and let T be the time of interaction. Note that S and T are known values. Suppose now that, during the interaction, the supports start moving from a standstill so that their acceleration remains non-negative all the time, and at the beginning and at the end of the movement their acceleration is zero. Note that during the interaction of the bar with the hips, the acceleration of the supports can be negative at no point, since otherwise the movement ceases to be supportive. We took a parabola as a model of such acceleration. If we take the starting time of the interaction as zero, then the form of this parabola is as follows: $y(t) = p \cdot t \cdot (T - t)$, where p is an unknown positive parameter, which is found from the condition that during time T the supports are shifted by value S. Then, given that the supports start moving from a standstill, we obtain:

$$a(t) = \frac{12 \cdot S}{T^4} t \cdot (T - t)$$

$$V(t) = \frac{12 \cdot S}{T^4} \left(\frac{T}{2} t^2 - \frac{t^3}{3} \right)$$

$$x(t) = \frac{12 \cdot S}{T^4} \left(\frac{T}{6} t^3 - \frac{t^4}{12} \right)$$

Here a(t), V(t) and x(t) are acceleration, velocity and displacement of the supports at moment t, respectively. The path of the support when repulsing the bar amounted to 3.39 cm. According to formula (5), we can now calculate the coordinates, speed and acceleration of the centers of weight masses as functions of time and, respectively, find the values of the horizontal force acting on the weight when repulsing the barbell by the hips (Fig. 7).

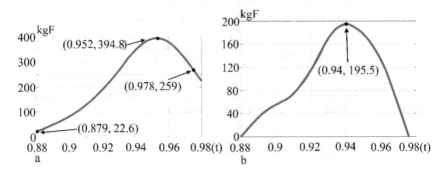

Fig. 7. Vertical (a) and horizontal (b) forces in kgF, acting on the weight when repulsing the barbell by the hips

Note that Fig. 7 shows the forces acting on one weight of the barbell only. In reality, the athlete acts on the bar with a double force.

7   Conclusion

The characteristic curves of space-time, dynamic and kinematic properties of a barbell snatch received by us and presented in this paper as well as the analysis of a microstructure of snatch allow to draw the following conclusions.

1. Use of high-speed video recording and the modern software allowed us to estimate space-time characteristics of the motion of the athlete and sporting equipment with high accuracy that in turn gave us the chance to analyze a microstructure of snatch and reveal the characteristics which are authentically connected with success of approach.
2. The important indicator in many respects defining success of attempt of the athlete of high qualification is height of approach of a barbell which in successful attempts is on average 0.02 m more, than in unsuccessful ones.
3. The liftoff size grows with increase in force of a repulse. In the given example due to a repulse the height of the barbell liftoff increases by 0.069 m [7].
4. From schedule 3 (b) – horizontal acceleration of a bar – it is possible to find time of interaction of the athlete with a bar during a repulse.

References

1. Burdett, R.G.: Biomechanics of the snatch technique of highly skilled and skilled weightlifters. Res. Q. Exerc. Sport **52**(3), 193–197 (1982)
2. Chiu, H.-T., Wang, C.-H., Cheng, K.B.: The three-dimensional kinematics of a barbell during the snatch of Taiwanese weightlifters. J. Strength Cond. Res. **24**(6), 1520–1526 (2010)
3. Lauder, M.A., Lake, J.P.: Biomechanical comparison of unilateral and bilateral power snatch lifts. J. Strength Cond. Res. **22**(3), 653–660 (2008)
4. Khasin, L.A.: Biomechanical analysis of weightlifter during classic jerk based on high-speed video recording and computer simulation. Theory Pract. Phys. Cult. (11), 100–104 (2013). (in Russian)
5. Khasin, L.A.: The biomechanical analysis of technology of performance of snatch by modern weightlifters of high qualification with use of high-speed video filming and mathematical modeling. Sports Sci. Bull. (1), 13–19 (2017). (in Russian)
6. Khasin, L.A., Burjan, S.B.: Calculation of horizontal forces applied by the athlete to the barbell when performing a snatch using high-speed video shooting and mathematical modeling. Theory Pract. Phys. Cult. **972**(6), 29–31 (2019). (in print, in Russian)
7. Khasin, L.A., Rafalovich, A.B., Androsov, P.I.: The comparative analysis of time-space characteristics of snatch of a bar in successful and unsuccessful attempts of weight-lifters of high qualification. Scientific Theory Journal "Uchenye zapiski universiteta imeni P.F. Lesgafta" **165**(11), 386–391 (2018). (in Russian)
8. Khasin, L.A., Drozdov, A.L.: Technique and results of the analysis of the technology of classical snatch performance. Scientific Theory Journal "Uchenye zapiski universiteta imeni P.F. Lesgafta" **165**(11), 382–386 (2018). (in Russian)

Evaluation of Foot Kinematics During Endurance Running on Different Surfaces in Real-World Environments

Markus Zrenner[1], Christoph Feldner[1], Ulf Jensen[2], Nils Roth[1(✉)], Robert Richer[1], and Bjoern M. Eskofier[1]

[1] Machine Learning and Data Analytics Lab, Friedrich-Alexander-Universität Erlangen-Nürnberg (FAU), Erlangen, Germany
{markus.zrenner,christoph.feldner,nils.roth,robert.richer, bjoern.eskofier}@fau.de
[2] Finance & IT – IT Innovation, adidas AG, Herzogenaurach, Germany
ulf.jensen@adidas.com

Abstract. Despite the fact that endurance running is an outdoor sport, most studies regarding foot kinematics have been conducted indoors in laboratories due to the stationary measurement equipment. Small and low-cost inertial measurement units (IMU) have proven to be accurate measurement tools for foot kinematics. In this study, we used such IMUs to evaluate the effect of different running surfaces on foot kinematics in a real-world scenario. For data collection, twenty amateur runners ran for at least one kilometer on six different surfaces, which were asphalt, tartan, gravel, bark mulch, grass and trail. From the acquired IMU data, we computed the sole angle, the maximum sole angle velocity, the range of motion in the frontal plane and the maximum pronation velocity for each stride. The results showed that the maximum angular rates as well as the absolute rotations are higher for stiffer and more consistent surfaces like tartan and asphalt.

Keywords: Wearable sensors · Inertial measurement units · Running · Terrain · Foot kinematics

1 Introduction

Endurance running is very popular and the reasons for its popularity are manifold: running is healthy [1], it has no restrictions to time and location and it has a low entrance barrier, because not much equipment is needed.

Due to these facts, a lot of research in running biomechanics has been conducted over the last decades with different foci like running shoe design [2], running economy [3] and injury prevention [4]. Over the years, different technologies have been developed and used to evaluate biomechanical parameters. In the beginning video cameras were used and the footage was labeled manually. Nowadays, marker based or marker less motion capture systems in combination

© Springer Nature Switzerland AG 2020
M. Lames et al. (Eds.): IACSS 2019, AISC 1028, pp. 106–113, 2020.
https://doi.org/10.1007/978-3-030-35048-2_13

with force plates became the gold standard, which can accurately determine kinetic as well as kinematic running parameters [5]. Despite the high accuracy, those systems have one drawback: they are stationary. Due to this fact most of the running related research was conducted within laboratories, even though running is an outdoor sport.

In recent years, many wearable systems were developed to overcome this discrepancy. Apart from other systems like insoles capable of measuring plantar pressure distributions during running, 6D inertial measurement units (IMUs) are a promising tool for the evaluation of various running related parameters. IMUs measure accelerations and angular rates and can easily be attached to the human body due to their small size. Strohrmann et al. [6] showed different applications for IMUs in running like skill level assessment, fatigue monitoring and training assistance by determining the foot contact duration, the foot strike type and the heel lift.

One kinematic parameter which has proven to have an impact on running kinematics is the surface runners run on. Hardin et al. showed that runners adapt to stiffer surfaces with increased peak angular velocities of the hip, knee, and ankle [7]. For their study, data was acquired on a treadmill with modifiable bed compliance so that different surfaces were only mimiced. Schuldhaus et al. [8] used IMUs to classify the surface on data of endurance runners that performed outdoor workouts. Their results showed that the movement patterns of runners change on different surfaces. However, the features that were used to classify the surface were very generic and can not be related to kinematic parameters.

In this work, we want to combine the approaches of Hardin et al. and Schuldhaus et al. by measuring interpretable foot kinematic parameters of runs in real-world environments. Therefore, we conducted a study with 20 subjects running on six different surfaces while wearing running shoes equipped with IMUs. The kinematic parameters for the evaluation are the sole angle, the maximum sole angle velocity, the range of motion in the frontal plane and the maximum pronation velocity.

2   Methods

2.1   Data Acquisition

We collected data of 20 amateur runners (11 male, 9 female). All subjects were informed about related risks and gave written consent to participate in the study and for the collected data to be published.[1] During data acquisition, the subjects wore a pair of running shoes (adidas Response Cushion 21, adidas AG, Herzogenaurach, Germany) which were equipped with 6D inertial measurement units (IMU) including a 3D-accelerometer and a 3D-gyroscope called miPod [9]. Data were sampled with 200 Hz with a resolution of 16 bit. The range of the accelerometer was ±16 g and the range of the gyroscope was ±2000 deg/s.

---

[1] The study was approved by the ethics committee of the Friedrich-Alexander-University Erlangen-Nürnberg, No. 106_13B.

The two sensors were located unobtrusively in a cavity in the insole of each running shoe. Before the data acquisition the sensors were calibrated using an approach introduced by Feraris et al. [10]. All subjects ran on a predefined track including six different surfaces: asphalt, tartan, gravel, bark mulch, grass and trail in a forest (Fig. 1). Within the different surfaces, the path was always flat and had no inclination. To prevent the effect of fatigue influencing the results, the first surface was randomly assigned for each subject. Afterwards the order of surfaces on which the subjects ran remained the same. The distance covered on each surface was at least 1 km. In total 154496 stride were collected for the evaluation of the kinematic parameters.

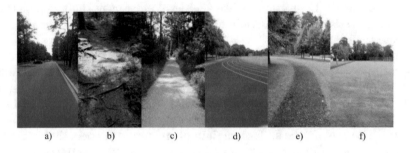

Fig. 1. Visualization of the different surfaces the subjects ran on during the data acquisition. (a) Asphalt, (b) Trail, (c) Gravel, (d) Tartan, (e) Bark Mulch, (f) Grass

2.2   Definition of Kinematic Parameters

The kinematic parameters that were used to evaluate the effect of the different surfaces were two angular and two angular rate parameters. The sole angle describes the angle between the sole of the running shoe and the ground during initial ground contact (IC) (Fig. 2). The range of motion describes the difference of the maximum eversion angle of the foot during stance phase and the inversion angle during the IC in the frontal plane (Fig. 2). The maximum sole angle velocity is the maximum angular rate during ground contact in the sagittal plane, whereas the maximum pronation velocity is the maximum angular rate during ground contact in the frontal plane.

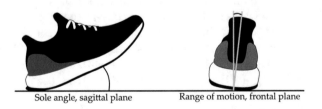

Fig. 2. Visualization of the kinematic parameters.

2.3 Data Processing

The data processing pipeline consisted of two steps: stride segmentation and kinematic parameter computation. It was previously introduced [11] and will thus only be briefly summarized. The algorithm used to segment single strides from the continuous IMU data stream is based on a threshold approach which finds acceleration peaks in dorsoventral direction during the IC. To prevent false positive detections of ICs, the segmentation algorithms searches for the swing phase prior to the distinctive peak caused by the IC impact.

If an IC is detected, the kinematic parameters from the gyroscope signals in the frontal and sagittal plane in a 250 ms window after the IC were computed. The duration of the window was defined to be 250 ms due to the fact, that this is the average duration of a stance phase while running with speeds up to 6 m/s [12]. The maximum sole angle velocity and the maximum pronation velocity can be computed be finding the maximum of the angular rate measured by the gyroscope in the sagittal and the frontal plane respectively. For the computation of the other two parameters the gyroscope signal was integrated in the 250 ms window to obtain angle values from the measured angular rate. For the integration process, the angle at IC was initialized with zero. The range of motion in frontal plane was determined by finding the maximum of the angle in the 250 ms window. The sole angle was computed by finding the minimum in the gyroscopic energy in the 250 ms after the IC, which is a common approach to determine the midstance phase in gait and running [13]. Thus, the angle value in the sagittal plane at this point in time describes the angle, that the foot rotated from the IC to midstance. Figure 3 depicts the described pipeline with exemplary data of one subject which participated in the study.

2.4 Evaluation

Due to the fact that the kinematic parameters differ for individual subjects, the kinematic parameters were normalized to observe differences among the surfaces. We normalized the kinematic parameters of each individual subject using z-score normalization [14]. The mean and standard deviation for the computation of the z-sore were determined over all different surfaces. After the normalization of the kinematic parameters we computed the mean value for all different surfaces. Thus, we obtain one z-score normalized mean value for each surface and each subject.

3 Results

Figure 4 depicts the results of the z-score normalized mean value of the maximum pronation velocity for the six different surfaces. One line represents the data of one subject. The plot indicates that the maximum pronation velocity is higher for the first three surfaces (aphalt, tartan, gravel), even though different subjects react differently to surface changes. For example, the maximum

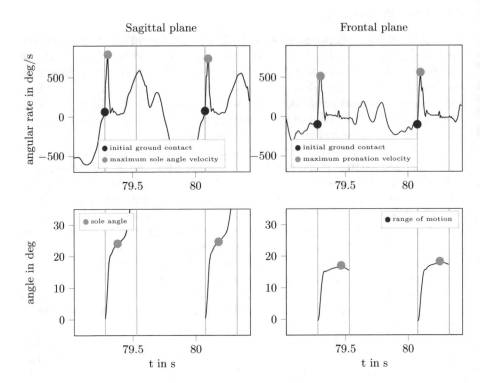

Fig. 3. Angular rate and angle data in sagittal and frontal plane over time for two exemplary strides. The red dots in the angular rate plots visualize the ICs determined by the stride segmentation algorithm. The violet vertical line depict the 250 ms window, in which the parameters are calculated. The green dots mark the parameters computed from the individual signals.

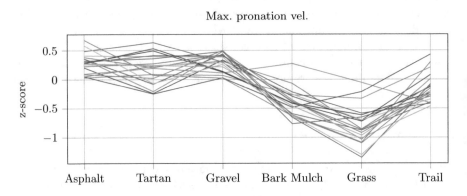

Fig. 4. Mean z-score of the maximum proantion velocity of the twenty subjects for six different surfacess. Each line represents one subject.

pronation velocity increases on tartan for some subjects (compared to asphalt or gravel), whereas it decreases for others.

Figure 5 visualizes the results for all kinematic parameters. One box represents one kinematic parameter on one surface for all twenty subjects. The results show that both the angular parameters (sole angle, range of motion) and the angular rate parameters (maximum sole angle velocity, maximum pronation velocity) are higher for stiffer and more consistent surfaces like asphalt or tartan than for less stiff and less consistent surfaces like grass or trail. When comparing the sole angle and the range of motion we observe that the angle differences in the sagittal plane are higher for the different surfaces than in the frontal plane. For some kinematic parameters the whiskers, indicating the range of the individual parameters on different surfaces, show that not all subjects react to surface changes in the same way. Due to the differences in physical conditions between male and female participants, we also evaluated the results for each gender individually. The trends in the differences we observed for the kinematic parameters were the same as the differences of the combined analysis presented in Fig. 5. Both males and females reacted to stiffer and more regular surfaces with increased angular and angular rate foot kinematics.

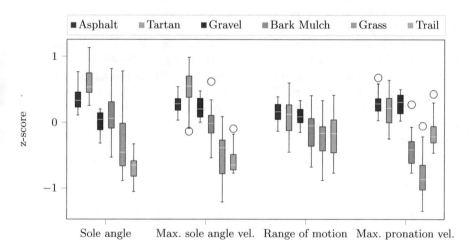

Fig. 5. Differences of maximum sole angle velocity for six different surfaces. The colored boxes visualize the upper and lower quartiles. The white line represents the median. The whiskers extend to 1.5 · IQR (interquartile range). The circles depict outliers. The surfaces are color coded. From left to right: asphalt (blue), tartan (grey), gravel (red), bark mulch (green), grass (green), trail (green).

4   Discussion

The results show that the kinematic parameters sole angle, maximum sole angle velocity, range of motion in the frontal plane and maximum pronation velocity change on different surfaces. We observe that the results of Hardin et al. [7] also hold for runs in real-world environments. Running on stiffer surfaces resulted in higher angular rates and higher absolute angles of the foot during ground contact. Hardin et al. [7] argued that these changes happen due to energy optimizations. Without adapting the initial ground contact angles, runners would have to flex their knee greater, which would result in a higher energy demand for weight support and push-off. One difference in our study was that not only the stiffness of the surfaces changed, but also the consistency. Asphalt and tartan are very flat surfaces, whereas the soil under grass can be uneven and roots sticking out of a trail are also obstacles during running. These different surface profiles might also influence the running kinematics, because runners will be more cautious to prevent themselves from twisting their ankles on softer and more uneven surfaces.

For some kinematic parameters on some surfaces, the whiskers indicating the parameter range and the outliers show that not all subjects in the study react to different surfaces in the same way. Thus, a classification of the surface using the four kinematic parameters considered in this work is not possible.

Even though we acquired data from real runs in a real-world environment, we still only evaluated data of one predefined running track, which included the different surfaces. During the data acquisition the weather conditions were always dry. The results presented in this work might change in case of rain and thus changing surface conditions. For example, tartan tracks get slippery when wet, which presumably effects foot kinematics. Future work shall tackle this by acquiring more data in other weather conditions. Besides, the proposed IMU based foot kinematics system could help to evaluate the effect of different shoe types on foot kinematics. Track shoes provide significantly more support and prevent runners from twisting their ankle. A study to evaluate whether changes in kinematics due to changes in footwear might be of interest for shoe manufacturers.

5   Conclusion

We conclude that kinematic parameter change on different surfaces during running. Stiffer and more regular surfaces like asphalt and tartan yield higher angular rates and higher foot rotations. This work also proves that IMUs are well suited to take kinematic parameter research from restricted indoor laboratories to runs in real-world environments. Using the proposed IMU-based system, further effects on running foot kinematics like surface changes due to changing weather conditions or different footwear can be evaluated in real-world running environments.

Acknowledgements. Bjoern Eskofier gratefully acknowledges the support of the German Research Foundation (DFG) within the framework of the Heisenberg professorship programme (grant 526 number ES 434/8-1).

References

1. Lee, D.-C., Pate, R.R., Lavie, C.J., Sui, X., Church, T.S., Blair, S.N.: Leisure-time running reduces all-cause and cardiovascular mortality risk. J. Am. Coll. Cardiol. **64**(5), 472–481 (2014)

2. Hoogkamer, W., Kipp, S., Frank, J.H., Farina, E.M., Luo, G., Kram, R.: A comparison of the energetic cost of running in marathon racing shoes. Sports Med. **48**(4), 1009–1019 (2018)

3. Anderson, T.: Biomechanics and running economy. Sports Med. **22**(2), 76–89 (1996)

4. Orchard, J.W., Fricker, P.A., Abud, A.T., Mason, B.R.: Biomechanics of iliotibial band friction syndrome in runners. Am. J. Sports Med. **24**(3), 375–379 (1996)

5. Colyer, S.L., Evans, M., Cosker, D.P., Salo, A.I.T.: A review of the evolution of vision-based motion analysis and the integration of advanced computer vision methods towards developing a markerless system. Sports Med.-Open **4**(1), 24 (2018)

6. Strohrmann, C., Harms, H., Tröster, G., Hensler, S., Müller, R.: Out of the lab and into the woods: kinematic analysis in running using wearable sensors. In: Proceedings of the 13 Annual Conference Ubiquitous Computing, pp. 119–122. ACM (2011)

7. Hardin, E.C., Den Bogert, A.J.V., Hamill, J.: Kinematic adaptations during running: effects of footwear surface and duration. Med. Sci. Sports Exerc. **36**(5), 838–844 (2004)

8. Schuldhaus, D., Kugler, P., Jensenm, U., Eskofier, B., Schlarb, H., Leible, M.: Classification of surfaces and inclinations during outdoor running using shoe-mounted inertial sensors. In: 21st ICPR, pp. 2258–2261. IEEE (2012)

9. Blank, P., Kugler, P., Schlarb, H., Eskofier, B.: A wearable sensor system for sports and fitness applications. In: 19th Annual Conference of the ECSS (2014)

10. Ferraris, F., Grimaldi, U., Parvis, M.: Procedure for effortless in-field calibration of three-axial rate gyro and accelerometers. Sens. Mat. **7**(5), 311–330 (1995)

11. Zrenner, M., Ullrich, M., Zobel, P., Jensen, U., Laser, F., Groh, B.H., Duemler, B., Eskofier, B.H.: Kinematic parameter evaluation for the purpose of a wearable running shoe recommendation. In: IEEE Transition BSN (2018)

12. De Wit, B., De Clercq, D., Aerts, P.: Biomechanical analysis of the stance phase during barefoot and shod running. J. Biomech. **33**(3), 269–278 (2000)

13. Skog, I., Handel, P., Nilsson, J.-O., Rantakokko, J.: Zero-velocity detection–an algorithm evaluation. IEEE Trans. Biomed. Eng. **57**(11), 2657–2666 (2010)

14. Larsen, R.J., Marx, M.L.: An Introduction to Mathematical Statistics and its Applications, vol. 2. Prentice-Hall Englewood Cliffs, New Jersey (1986)

Unobtrusive Estimation of In-Stroke Boat Rotation in Rowing Using Wearable Sensors

Benjamin H. Groh[1]([⊠]), Julia Schottenhamml[1], Bjoern M. Eskofier[1], and Ami Drory[2]

[1] Machine Learning and Data Analytics Lab, Department of Computer Science, Friedrich-Alexander-Universität Erlangen-Nürnberg (FAU), Erlangen, Germany
benjamin.groh@fau.de
[2] Bioengineering Research Group, Faculty of Engineering, University of Nottingham, Nottingham, UK

Abstract. The rotational motion of a rowing boat during single strokes has significant impact on the boat velocity and overall rowing performance. However, a method for automatic in-stroke field quantification remains challenging. In this work, we propose a robust stroke segmentation algorithm in combination with a 3D-rotation estimation during segmented strokes. Our method is designed to process unobtrusively obtained inertial sensor data of one sensor device attached to rowing boats. A template-based matching algorithm is implemented to detect all strokes in the collected sensor data. The segmented strokes are then analyzed for the corresponding in-stroke rotation. The evaluation of the stroke segmentation was performed with professional race and amateur training data. The resulting precision was 99.8 % for professional and 97.2 % for amateur data. The in-stroke rotation angle calculation was validated with amateur training data of four boat classes. The results were compared to corresponding measurements from the literature.

Keywords: Inertial sensing · Rowing · Template-based segmentation · 3D-rotation estimation

1 Introduction

The rotational motion of a rowing boat has significant impact on the boat velocity and rowing performance. It is often used as an indirect performance measure of rowing technique [9]. Whilst this performance measure is routinely qualitatively assessed by coaches, its in-field quantification remains challenging. Hence, a solution that provides continuous analysis of the boat motion will constitute a powerful indicator for technique and performance evaluation.

Continuous analysis could be achieved by the application of wearable inertial sensors, containing 3D-accelerometers and 3D-gyroscopes. State-of-the-art algorithms provide rotation estimation of inertial measurement units (IMUs).

© Springer Nature Switzerland AG 2020
M. Lames et al. (Eds.): IACSS 2019, AISC 1028, pp. 114–122, 2020.
https://doi.org/10.1007/978-3-030-35048-2_14

By attaching an IMU to a rowing boat, the continuous rotation could be monitored and processed to an indicator for technique and performance evaluation.

It has to be considered that this evaluation would not be focused on the overall rotation but rather on the rotation during single rowing strokes. Hence, a stroke segmentation method is required before calculating the in-stroke rotation. In order to avoid additional measurements, the stroke segmentation could be based on the obtained IMU data. The resulting algorithm would be a combined solution of an IMU-based stroke segmentation with a subsequent in-stroke rotation calculation. Such an approach could even be automated for enhanced race and training analysis.

Rowing technique has been extensively analyzed over the past decade. The boat's rotation was of special interest for the boat's motion asymmetry [10] and for the boat's stability with the aim of reducing the athletes' motion effort [3,9]. However, only few publications focused on the topic of rotation estimation. Wagner et al. [12] first proposed measurements with gyroscopes in a single scull boat. Loschner et al. [5] followed up on this approach and obtained the 3D-orientation of single scull boats. Gravenhorst et al. [3] computed the angular velocity of the motion but did not calculate corresponding angles. Sinclair et al. [9] estimated the in-stroke boat rotation by processing the vertical and horizontal displacement. Serveto et al. [8] calculated the boat's pitch angle and compared it to accelerometer measurements.

The aforementioned publications focused on only few boat classes instead of including a larger variety. Furthermore, they did not provide any stroke segmentation, which would be necessary for an automated analysis. The only known IMU-based rowing stroke segmentation was presented by previous work of our group [4]. Acceleration data were obtained from professional rowing races and processed by a continuous stroke segmentation algorithm.

In this work, we extend the previously published stroke segmentation by an evaluation with professional race and amateur training data. Furthermore, we propose a combined algorithm for stroke segmentation and subsequent 3D-rotation calculation. The results of the determined boat rotation angles are compared to values from the literature.

2   Methods

2.1   Data Acquisition

The data acquisition was divided into two parts: for data from professional athletes during competition (referred to as 'professional data') and for data from amateur participants during training (referred to as 'amateur data'). The goal was to use professional data for the evaluation of the stroke segmentation and to use amateur data for both the evaluation of the stroke segmentation and the calculation of the in-stroke rotation.

Hardware. The sensor hardware for collecting professional data consisted of the three-axes accelerometer Analog Devices ADXL330. The sensor was integrated in the on-board tracking unit, which is mounted to all rowing boats in most professional contests. The accelerometer was configured to a range of $\pm 3\,g$ and provided data with a sampling rate of 50 Hz.

For collecting the amateur data during training, the miPod IMU [2] (containing an Invensense MPU-9150 sensor) was used. Its ranges were set to $\pm 8\,g$ (accelerometer) and $\pm 1000\,°/s$ (gyroscope) with a sampling rate of 200 Hz. One unit was attached per boat. It was mounted in the boat's cavity, as shown in Fig. 1.

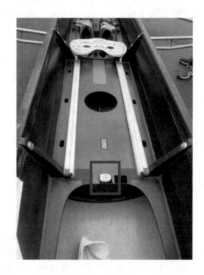

Fig. 1. Attachment of the miPod IMU inside the boat cavity.

Study Design. The professional rowing data were collected during the U23 World Championship 2013 on the regatta course of Linz-Ottensheim, Austria. The focus was set on two boat classes (1x: single scull and 8+: coxed eight), which were assumed to represent the extrema of all race boat classes in size, velocity and general motion behavior. Data of multiple races in these classes were collected, including heat, repechage, semi-finals and finals for both male and female athletes. An overview of all data sets with the corresponding boat class and number of rowing strokes is presented in Table 1.

The amateur rowing data were collected during training on the Rems river in Waiblingen, Germany. The focus was set on four boat classes (1x: single scull, 2x: double scull, 4x: quadruple scull, 8+: eight coxed) with up to nine participants. Multiple rowing intervals with a duration between 20 s and 60 s were recorded. Four intervals per boat class were selected for further processing. An overview of all data sets with corresponding boat class and the total number of rowing strokes (for all four intervals) is presented in Table 1.

For the acquisition with amateur athletes, a sensor calibration was performed before the training started. This included static positions of the IMU on each of the six sides for accelerometer calibration and defined rotations about all three axes individually for gyroscope calibration. For the acquisition with professional athletes, no sensor calibration was performed in order to avoid interruptions in the contest procedure.

Table 1. Overview of professional (P) and amateur (A) data sets, including boat class, type of race (only for professional data) and number of strokes.

ID	boat class	race type	strokes
	professional: single scull		
P1	lightweight, women (LW1x)	heat	247
P2	men (M1x)	repechage	246
P3	lightweight, men (LM1x)	quarter final	221
P4	women (W1x)	semi final	265
P5	lightweight, women (LW1x)	final	277
P6	men (M1x)	final	227
	professional: coxed eight		
P7	men (M8+)	heat	223
P8	women (W8+)	repechage	240
P9	women (W8+)	final	257
P10	men (M8+)	final	222
	amateur		
A1	single scull, men (M1x)	–	48
A2	double scull, men (M2x)	–	54
A3	quadruple scull, men (M4x)	–	39
A4	coxed eight, mixed (M/W8+)	–	38

2.2   Template-Based Rowing Stroke Segmentation

The segmentation of rowing strokes was performed with dynamic time warping (DTW) [1], a template-based matching algorithm. By defining the template to represent one rowing stroke, DTW provided the recognition of similar strokes in a corresponding signal. In order to obtain multiple results of consecutive strokes instead of the recognition of only one stroke, an extension for continuous template matching was applied: subsequent dynamic time warping (subDTW) [6]. The approach of applying subDTW to rowing strokes was based on our previous work in [4]. Although the rowing motion is of interest in three dimensions, the processing of only the 1D-acceleration signal in motion direction led to robust segmentation results and thus, also the segmentation approach of this work was based on the 1D-acceleration in motion direction.

Strokes were defined to start and end at the highest negative acceleration, i.e., between catch phase and drive phase [11] (see Fig. 2). The template was randomly and manually selected from the continuous acceleration signal. Before applying subDTW, both template and signal were lowpass filtered with a moving average (span: 0.4 s). Furthermore, the algorithm was adapted to suit rowing-specific requirements by including a minimum stroke duration of 0.8 s.

2.3   In-Stroke Rotation Calculation

The segmented strokes of the amateur data sets were further processed for the in-stroke rotation calculation. This computation was based on the 3D-gyroscope signal. The angular rate $\boldsymbol{\omega}$ of each segmented stroke was processed with a quaternion-based integration method. Assuming constant sampling frequency f, the rotation magnitude Ω_t and the rotation vector $\boldsymbol{v}_t$ were calculated for each sampling step t (see Eq. 1). Both were further processed to the corresponding quaternion $\boldsymbol{q}_t$ (see Eq. 2). The overall in-stroke rotation was then computed by multiplication of consecutive quaternions [7]. For reasons of later evaluation, the resulting overall quaternion per stroke was transformed to Euler angles (yaw, pitch, roll).

$$\Omega_t = \frac{1}{f} \cdot \left\|\boldsymbol{\omega}_t\right\|_2 \qquad \boldsymbol{v}_t = \frac{\boldsymbol{\omega}_t}{\left\|\boldsymbol{\omega}_t\right\|_2} \tag{1}$$

$$\boldsymbol{q}_t = \begin{bmatrix} \cos(\frac{\Omega_t}{2}) \\ v_t^{\mathrm{x}} \cdot \sin(\frac{\Omega_t}{2}) \\ v_t^{\mathrm{y}} \cdot \sin(\frac{\Omega_t}{2}) \\ v_t^{\mathrm{z}} \cdot \sin(\frac{\Omega_t}{2}) \end{bmatrix} \tag{2}$$

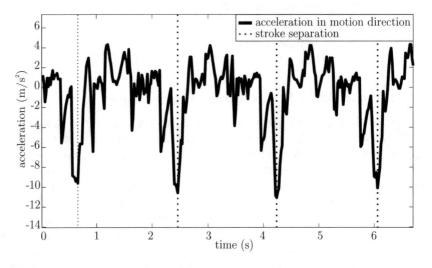

Fig. 2. Acceleration signal of consecutive rowing strokes (from P5: LW1x, final). The dotted lines indicate the defined separation between strokes.

2.4   Evaluation

Rowing Stroke Segmentation. The stroke segmentation was evaluated with both professional and amateur data. However, templates were only extracted from professional data to analyze both the segmentation of race data templates with race data signals and the segmentation of race data templates with training data signals.

From each of the ten professional data sets, one template was extracted. All ten templates were then applied to all ten professional data sets and additionally, to all four amateur data sets (see Table 1). The precision and recall were calculated for all combinations and averaged for all professional and all amateur data sets.

Rotation Calculation. The resulting in-stroke rotation angles were compared to three publications from the literature. Loschner et al. [5] published their 3D-gyroscope-based rotation angles based on data from elite level athletes in single scull boats. Sinclair et al. [9] provided their findings on single scull boat rotation for advanced to elite level athletes by means of horizontal and vertical displacement. For the evaluation of this work, the displacement was transformed to corresponding Euler angles, assuming an average boat length of 8.2 m and an estimated distance between oar locks of 1.6 m. Serveto et al. [8] presented accelerometer-based measurements of the pitch angle. An overview of these literature values is presented in Table 2.

The angular rotation calculation of all strokes were combined per boat class and additionally averaged over all data sets. The results are presented by the overall range (minimum and maximum values) and the mean and standard deviation.

Table 2. Literature values vs. results of this work for angular boat rotation angles.

source	details	boat rotation angles		
		yaw	pitch	roll
Loschner et al. [5]	gyroscope data, elite level, 13 single scull athletes	0.5°	0.2°	1.7°
Sinclair et al. [9]	boat displacement, adv. to elite level, 11 single scull athletes	0.04°	0.28°	0.36°
Serveto et al. [8]	accelerometer data	–	0.73°	–
results of this work (see Table 3)	gyroscope data, amateur level, four boat classes	0.92°	0.48°	2.43°

3   Results

3.1   Rowing Stroke Segmentation.

The segmentation results for professional data sets showed an overall precision of 0.998 and an overall recall of 0.997. For the amateur data sets (processed with templates from the professional data sets) the overall precision and recall were evaluated to 0.972 and 0.904.

3.2   Rotation Calculation.

The resulting in-stroke angles for all boat classes are presented in Table 3 with their range, mean and standard deviation. The overall mean and standard deviation over all four boat classes were computed to be $0.92° \pm 0.92°$ (yaw), $0.48° \pm 0.11°$ (pitch) and $2.43° \pm 0.99°$ (roll).

Table 3. Results of the rotation calculation: in-stroke ranges for yaw, pitch and roll angles for all four amateur data sets.

ID	yaw range (°)		pitch range (°)		roll range (°)	
	min; max	mean ± std	min; max	mean ± std	min; max	mean ± std
A1	0.22; 7.17	0.97 ± 1.20	0.25; 0.73	0.45 ± 0.12	1.06; 4.41	2.31 ± 0.86
A2	0.15; 5.04	0.80 ± 0.83	0.41; 0.85	0.59 ± 0.09	1.38; 7.40	2.79 ± 1.27
A3	0.16; 2.89	0.92 ± 0.61	0.31; 0.73	0.52 ± 0.10	0.91; 4.40	2.22 ± 0.84
A4	0.18; 5.00	1.00 ± 0.94	0.20; 0.73	0.37 ± 0.14	0.94; 4.51	2.39 ± 0.91
		0.92 ± 0.92		**0.48 ± 0.11**		**2.43 ± 0.99**

4   Discussion

The results of the subDTW-based stroke segmentation showed that randomly selected templates from any boat class during professional races lead to robust segmentation for all obtained professional race data. With accuracies of over 99 % for both precision and recall, an accurate boat class-independent segmentation was achieved. Furthermore, the application of templates from professional data to signals from amateur data showed only slightly worse results with a precision of 97.2 % and a recall of 90.4 %.

The established rotation calculation showed similar ranges for all four boat classes. The calculated pitch angle coincides with values from the literature. Both the yaw and the roll angle show slightly increased rotation of the measured amateur data in comparison to the literature values. This could be explained by the difference in skill level between amateur athletes in this work and advanced to elite level athletes in the literature.

Improvements of the provided methods could be achieved by an advanced template creation. Instead of selecting random templates of race data from one boat class, more specifically adjusted templates could be built either per application scenario (competitions or training) or even per boat class. Furthermore, multiple strokes could be combined for the template creation to minimize the risk of unsuitable templates. Concerning the rotation calculation, improvements could be achieved by an enhanced sensor calibration and attachment. For the amateur data acquisition, the sensors were calibrated once before the training. However, the sensor output can slightly change due to temperature and acquisition duration. Furthermore, the sensor attachment was performed in a way that the sensor's coordinate system was visually aligned with the boat's axes. Due to the visual alignment, a slight deviation between sensor and boat system cannot be excluded.

Although the algorithm potentially could be improved by aforementioned modifications, the overall results indicate its robustness and applicability to competitions and training scenarios. Further applications of the provided algorithm could be achieved by a stroke rate calculation (based on the provided stroke segmentation) and an (automated) training feedback, e.g., by alerting the athletes of incorrect rowing performance, when defined rotation angles are exceeded.

5   Conclusion

In this work, a robust algorithm for the segmentation of continuous rowing strokes with subsequent in-stroke rotation calculation was presented. It can find its application in rowing competitions and training. The proposed algorithm provides the foundation for further development towards automated rowing performance feedback. In addition, future work could include further stroke- and in-stroke-related applications, such as a stroke rate estimation, which could directly be derived from the proposed segmentation algorithm.

Acknowledgments. The authors would like to thank the rowing club Rudergesellschaft Ghibellinia Waiblingen for their participation in the data acquisition.

References

1. Berndt, D.J., Clifford, J.: Using dynamic time warping to find patterns in time series. In: KDD Workshop on Knowledge Discovery in Databases, pp. 359–370. AAAI (1994)
2. Blank, P., Kugler, P., Schlarb, H., Eskofier, B.: A wearable sensor system for sports and fitness applications. In: 19th Annual Conference of the European College of Sport Science, p. 703. ECSS (2014)
3. Gravenhorst, F., Tessendorf, B., Arnrich, B., Tröster, G.: Analyzing rowing crews in different rowing boats based on angular velocity measurements with gyroscopes. In: 8th International Symposium on Computer Science in Sport (IACSS), pp. 1–4. IACSS (2011)

4. Groh, B.H., Reinfelder, S.J., Streicher, M.N., Taraben, A., Eskofier, B.M.: Movement prediction in rowing using a dynamic time warping based stroke detection. In: 9th International Conference on Intelligent Sensors, Sensor Networks and Information Processing (ISSNIP), pp. 1–6. IEEE (2014)
5. Loschner, C., Smith, R., Galloway, M.: Intra-stroke boat orientation during single sculling. In: 18th International Symposium on Biomechanics in Sports, pp. 1–4. ISBS (2000)
6. Müller, M.: Dynamic time warping. Information Retrieval for Music and Motion, vol. 4, pp. 69–84. Springer, Berlin (2007)
7. Pujol, J.: Hamilton, Rodrigues, Gauss, quaternions, and rotations: a historical reassessment. Commun. Math. Anal. **13**(2), 1–14 (2012)
8. Serveto, S., Barré, S., Kobus, J.M., Mariot, J.P.: A three-dimensional model of the boat-oars-rower system using ADAMS and LifeMOD commercial software. Proc. Inst. Mech. Eng., Part P: J. Sports Eng. Technol. **224**(1), 75–88 (2010)
9. Sinclair, P.J., Greene, A.J., Smith, R.: The effects of horizontal and vertical forces on single scull boat orientation while rowing. In: 27th International Conference on Biomechanics in Sports, pp. 1–4. ISBS (2009)
10. Smith, R., Draper, C.: Quantitative characteristics of coxless pair-oar rowing. In: 20th International Symposium on Biomechanics in Sports, pp. 263–266. ISBS (2002)
11. Tessendorf, B., Gravenhorst, F., Arnrich, B., Tröster, G.: An IMU-based sensor network to continuously monitor rowing technique on the water. In: 7th International Conference on Intelligent Sensors, Sensor Networks and Information Processing (ISSNIP), pp. 253–258. IEEE (2011)
12. Wagner, J., Bartmus, U., De Marees, H.: Three-axes gyro system quantifying the specific balance of rowing. Int. J. Sports Med. **14**(S1), S35–S38 (1993)

Probabilistic Performance Profiling

A Model of the Power Duration Relation in Endurance Sports

Alexander Asteroth[✉], Melanie Ludwig, and Kevin Bach

Bonn-Rhein-Sieg University o.A.S., Sankt Augustin, Germany
`alexander.asteroth@h-brs.de`

Abstract. A probabilistic model of maximal mean performance in endurance sports is presented. The joint distribution of three variables namely interval length, average power, and average heart rate is modeled using Gaussian processes. The model allows for prediction of maximal average performances even based on data from sub-maximal efforts.

Keywords: Critical power · Probabilistic model · Gaussian processes · Performance profiling

1 Introduction

The power-duration relation has been studied thoroughly during the last century. If a constant workload P is applied, time to fatigue T_{lim} can be observed. As early as the 1920s, physiological aspects [9] were the focus of A.V. Hill and other's research. Later, focus shifted to threshold concepts that were studied by Monod and Scherrer [12] on the level of small muscle groups, up to the level of total body work by Moritani et al. [13]. The discovery of asymptotic relation [12,13] between time to exhaustion T_{lim} and power P given as

$$(P - CP) \cdot T_{lim} = W' \tag{1}$$

made the asymptote (critical power, CP) a perfect candidate to be correlated with physiological thresholds [6,10,13]. Recently, with digital performance measurement becoming more and more common in endurance sports, focus has moved from characteristic parameters of the curve towards considering its complete shape [7,8,14,16]. Digital recording of power and speed data from whole competitions and training sessions allows for mean maximal performance (MMP) analysis yielding a power/speed-duration curve for a particular event, or even a whole season. Such MMP data can be used to profile an athletic performance or the demand of a particular type of competition. It more and more replaces traditional heart rate based profiling [16] and training control. Recently, Karsten et al. have shown that MMP data can serve as a basis to reliably compute CP [11].

While CP was successfully correlated to different physiological thresholds in the 80s and 90s, later studies indicate that CP does not represent a proper

© Springer Nature Switzerland AG 2020
M. Lames et al. (Eds.): IACSS 2019, AISC 1028, pp. 123–131, 2020.
https://doi.org/10.1007/978-3-030-35048-2_15

threshold in itself since lactate values continually increased at work at CP-level [3]. T_{lim} at CP has shown to be only around 20 min on average and varies significantly between test subjects [3]. This leads to the conclusion that the asymptotic relation of the CP-model significantly overestimates T_{lim} for durations longer than 20 min. MMP data can provide a more realistic estimation of T_{lim} as it is based on measurements only, and since no extrapolation takes place performance cannot be overestimated. However, this only applies if all-out efforts for the considered duration are available in data. In the analyzes of Karsten et al. [11], it was possible to compute CP based on MMP either using a standardized field testing protocol or alternatively based on competition data (including max. efforts for 3, 7 and 12 min; similar to [14]).

Summarizing, MMP data provides more detailed information about the actual performance profile (PP) of an athlete than CP modeling alone. Moreover, it does not depend on laboratory all-out tests because it is based on data that is usually already available. The biggest weakness, however, is the systematic underestimation of an athlete's performance and thus the strong dependence on data quality.

2 Method

To overcome the shortcoming of MMP underestimating "true" maximal performance ($\widehat{P}$), we suggest a probabilistic approach that will lead to a probabilistic performance profile (PPP). The approach is based on Gaussian process regression (GP) to model the power-duration relation [15]. We will model the more general relation between power, heart rate and duration, and from this model we will extract the $\widehat{P}$-T_{lim} relation. We will use three random variables: duration T, average heart rate HR, and average power P to model an athlete's performance[1]. P marks the objective effort an athlete produces over some interval duration T, while HR can be seen as a marker for the subjective effort of this athletic performance. This allows objective and subjective effort to be linked in the PPP. In maximal performances, we assume both measures to be (almost) maximal at the same time. We do not expect a simple functional relation between these variables, as the complex physiological mechanisms influencing HR will be ignored by the model. Instead, the general idea is to model the joint distribution.

$$Prob(P = p, HR = hr, T = t) \tag{2}$$

using historic training data from which absolute frequencies of triples (P, HR, T) are determined. As an example, Fig. 1 shows one "slice" of this multidimensional data (data is described in more detail in Sect. 3), namely frequencies of ($HR, P, T = 360s$) for subject $P5$. Samples are generated using a moving average filter over data from the last T sec (in case of Fig. 1, window size is 360 as data sample rate is 1 Hz). For each training, the filter allows generation of

---

[1] In case of cycling power is available for measurement by means of power meters; in case of, e.g., running, power can be estimated by running speed.

a sample for every point within the interval $[T, N]$, with N being the size of the data set, thus resulting in a sufficient number of samples (369,896 samples in case of Fig. 1). The estimation of the probability densities is based on these frequency data.

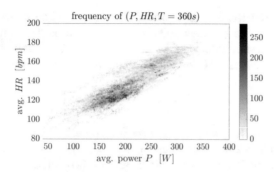

Fig. 1. Frequencies of $(HR, P, T = 360s)$ triples for subject $P5$ based on 369,896 samples generated from 20 training data sets.

We do not model the joint distribution directly but rather follow a multi-step process leading to the *PPP*, the probabilistic model of maximal average power $\widehat{P}$:

1. maximal heart rates $hr_{\max,t}$ are determined[2] from the sampled data;
2. by means of *GP* regression [15] (cf. Sect. 2.1), we can approximate

$$g(hr, p, t) = Prob(HR = hr \mid P = p, T = t), \tag{3}$$

3. and using Bayes' rule compute

$$f(p, hr, t) = Prob(P = p \mid HR = hr, T = t); \tag{4}$$

4. as we assume that $\widehat{P}$ occurs at maximal heart rate, we have

$$Prob(\widehat{P} = p \mid T = t) = f(p, hr_{\max,t}, t) \tag{5}$$

Main aspects of those steps are explained in detail in the following subsections.

2.1   Gaussian Process Regression

As we do not only want to interpolate the distribution of HR, but also extrapolate unknown values (we assume that only sub-maximal data is available), we use a Gaussian Process Model [15] to accomplish this task. *GP* models use a

---

[2] E.g. assuming a simple hyperbolic relation HR-T.

generalization of the Gaussian distribution: instead of describing random variables defined by mean and variance, a *GP* describes a random distribution of functions h defined by a mean function μ, and a covariance function k:

$$h(\mathbf{x}) \sim GP(\mu(\mathbf{x}), k(\mathbf{x}, \mathbf{x}')). \tag{6}$$

In our concrete case, $\mathbf{x} = (p, t)$ and $HR = h(p, t)$. The Covariance function k defines the relationship between neighboring values precisely in form of a kernel. Here we use a common choice of kernel, the squared exponential function. As points $\mathbf{x}$ become closer, their values get exponentially more correlated, so

$$k(\mathbf{x}_i, \mathbf{x}_j) = \exp\left(-\frac{1}{2}\|\mathbf{x}_i - \mathbf{x}_j\|^2\right). \tag{7}$$

Modeling $Prob(HR = hr \mid P = p, T = t)$ by means of a *GP* model can be seen as interpreting HR as a random function $hr = h(p, t)$. This function is distributed according to $g(hr, p, t)$ for known values, and extrapolated by Gaussian process regression otherwise. We know that the relation between the variables HR and P is approximately linear [1] for a given duration t up to the HR-deflection point [2,4,5], and that it will not exceed $hr_{\max,t}$. Therefore, instead of the usual choice of $\mu(\mathbf{x}) = 0$, a linear relation that is cut off at $hr_{\max,t}$ will be used as the prior mean value function of the GP model. It can be estimated by a linear regression based on the samples of $(HR, P, T = t)$ (cf. Fig. 2 (left)). From this prior distribution we now derive a posterior distribution given the set of observations $D = \{((p_i, t_i), hr_i) \mid i = 1, \ldots, n\}$ based on our training data. In this process, the mean function is adjusted to correspond to the actual mean at every observed point, and covariance is adjusted accordingly (for details about the posterior see, e.g., [15]). Figure 2 shows an example of both, the prior and the resulting posterior distribution for cyclist $P4$ season S_{42} (cf. Sect. 3).

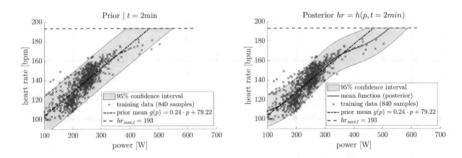

Fig. 2. (left) prior distribution of HR for $T = 2$ min. Linear mean function is estimated from data; (right) posterior distribution estimated by GP. It can be seen that GP is able to capture HR deflection.

2.2   Estimation of $\widehat{P}$

The Gaussian process posterior is now used to determine the density $g(hr, p, t)$ (Eq. (3)), from which by means of Bayes' rule we derive density $f(p, hr, t)$ (Eq. (4)). In a final step, we use the maximum estimated heart rate $hr_{\max,t}$ which leads to the distribution of $\widehat{P}$

$$Prob(\widehat{P} = p, T = t) = f(p, hr_{\max,t}, t) \tag{8}$$

Figure 3(left) shows an example of the resulting distribution of $\widehat{P}$. As can be seen, a distribution of maximal power outputs is predicted for every interval duration. The prediction is based on sub-maximal training only. Nevertheless, evaluation will show that prediction is quite accurate.

3   Evaluation

Experiments to evaluate the presented approach are based on training load data of five professional male cyclists collected over 22 weeks (April–September 2015). Daily training alternated between active recovery, competition training, endurance and tempo training. Data of performed competitions is included as well. Additional strength training of the athletes is not included in this analysis. In total, between 89 and 120 data-sets were available per athlete. Basic characteristics of the athletes are summarized in Table 1. We separated the data into sub-seasons (depending on data availability) to avoid comparison between data from beginning and end of a season. Sub-seasons were chosen to contain more than 12 data-sets that were non-competition sub-maximal trainings (NC). Within each sub-period, we separated NC-data that was used to train the *GP* model. Table 2 summarizes the data-sets used in the evaluation. For each subject and each period, a *PPP* was trained based on the corresponding training data and tested using all data (including competition data) from this same period. E.g., for cyclist P4 in sub-season S_{42}, 14 data sets were used to train the *PPP*.

Table 1. Characteristics of the cyclists who participated in this study

	P1	P2	P3	P4	P5
Age (at begin of the study)	21	20	18	19	21
Height [cm]	183	184	189	179	180
Weight [kg]	77.6 ± 0.7	75.4 ± 0.7	69.6 ± 0.6	76.9 ± 0.7	80.6 ± 0.5
Training load p.a. [km]	ca. 18,000	ca. 20,000	ca. 18,000	ca. 16,000	ca. 22,000

We decided to use the competition data as an estimate of *"true"* $\widehat{P}$. Real ground truth data would mean determination of T_{lim} for a huge number of power values – which obviously is unfeasible. As we were interested in determining true

Table 2. Data partitioning, each sub-season was chosen such that more than 12 NC-trainings were included. Numbers in brackets show (no. samples total/no. NC-samples)

Subject	4/2015	5/2015	6/2015	7/2015	8/2015	9/2015
P1	S_{11} (20/15)	S_{12} (41/23)	—		S_{13} (39/27)	
P2	S_{21} (21/14)	S_{22} (19/13)	S_{23} (40/18)		—	
P3	S_{31} (27/17)			S_{32} (33/19)		S_{33}(33/16)
P4	—	S_{41} (36/13)		S_{42} (23/14)		—
P5	S_{51} (19/15)	S_{52} (42/13)		—		—

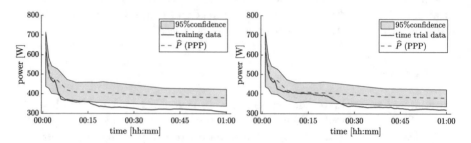

Fig. 3. (left) *MMP* of underlying data (*training data*) as well as $\widehat{P}$ predicted by *PPP* is shown. As can be seen prediction is considerably higher then input data; (right) probabilistic model of $\widehat{P}$ for athlete P4, season S_{42}. Model predicts MMP_{20} quite accurately even though it is trained on sub-maximal data only.

$\widehat{P}$ values, we included all available data for this sub-season. As an example, Fig. 3 (right) shows the experiment for season S_{42}.

Athlete P4 obviously did only all-out efforts up to 20 min, which included a 20 min "time trial". It can be seen that the probabilistic performance profile quite accurately predicted the maximal mean power that athlete P4 is able to sustain for 20 minutes, even though it is estimated from sub-maximal training only.

Results. For all 13 sub-seasons, a *PPP* was trained. The model then was used to predict observed *MMP* values for 11 different durations

$$T \in \{1', 2', 3', 5', 8', 11', 15', 18', 20', 40', 60'\}.$$

For each duration, the predicted mean was compared to the actual observed *MMP* in all data for this sub-season, and relative error

$$rd(a, b) = \frac{|a - b|}{b} \tag{9}$$

was recorded. On average, an error slightly above 5% was observed (median 0.057 with std.-dev. 0.067, see Fig. 4 (right)). The error varied for different durations, ranging from 0.042–0.085. 1 min was the hardest to predict, $2 - 11$ min are the durations that were best predicted (see Fig. 4 (left)). The median of prediction errors varied significantly between test subjects, from 0.026 for athlete P4 up to 0.165 for athlete P1 as can be seen in Table 3.

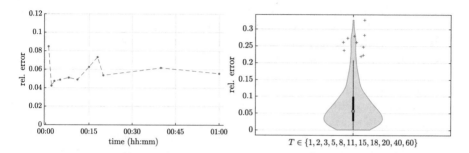

Fig. 4. (left) mean average relative errors $rd(\widehat{P}(t), MMP(t))$ is shown for all 11 durations for which the model was evaluated. For every duration, the mean was computed over all 13 sub-seasons; (right) distribution of error is shown as violin plot based on all 143 data points. About 25% of the errors are above 10%. Further analysis yields that this is mainly caused by data from test subject P1.

Table 3. Rel. error test athletes; median (std.-dev.) is shown for each sub-season (cf. 2).

Subject	Relative-error		
P1	S_{11}: 0.1552 (0.0903)	S_{12}: 0.2195 (0.0561)	S_{13}: 0.1196 (0.0265)
P2	S_{21}: 0.0572 (0.0276)	S_{22}: 0.0385 (0.0773)	S_{23}: 0.0489 (0.0262)
P3	S_{31}: 0.0635 (0.0531)	S_{32}: 0.0634 (0.0704)	S_{33}: 0.0490 (0.0392)
P4	S_{41}: 0.0359 (0.0168)	S_{42}: 0.0170 (0.0119)	
P5	S_{51}: 0.0476 (0.0352)	S_{52}: 0.0289 (0.0491)	

4   Discussion

An overall error of around 5% was achieved in evaluation. Since $HR\text{-}P$ relation is much noisier in case of 1 min durations, it is obvious that this leads to higher errors in a probabilistic model. A slight upward trend in the error towards longer durations can be explained by the fact that athletes do not regularly make all-out efforts for longer durations, thus the test data in this case does not correctly represent true $\widehat{P}$. Variation between test subjects was expected, but evaluation showed higher variability than anticipated. Apparently, the athletes' varying training habits influence outcome of the evaluation. Whether this is due to the quality of the test data or to the quality of the prediction by the PPP will be the subject of further research. As it cannot be assured, and indeed is unlikely that for all tested durations actual maximal MMP values are present in the test data, this is a significant source of error. The model will overestimate the observed value (just because observed MMP is not a maximal effort).

Derivation of the PPP used the assumption that mean maximal HR depends hyperbolically on duration. It would be preferable if this assumption did not have to be made since the approach generally does not need this assumption since $hr_{\max,t}$ could also be estimated using GP.

Initially, we assumed that the distribution $Prob(HR = hr \mid P = p, T = t)$ would exhibit an asymmetric shape, and as HR is bounded, also a distribution with finite support would be reasonable (e.g., an extreme value distribution). In the evaluation it turned out that the prediction worked well even with a GP using a normal distribution. Due to averaging, the distribution of HR seemed approximately Gaussian.

Furthermore, the evaluation showed that prediction works better for some athletes than for others. Future work will investigate whether this is caused by the method or by the evaluation strategy using data from more athletes. Summarizing, the approach seems to be a very promising extension to the classical CP concept and MMP analyses.

References

1. Arts, F., Kuipers, H.: The relation between power output, oxygen uptake and heart rate in male athletes. Int. J. Sports Med. **15**(05), 228–231 (1994)
2. Bodner, M.E., Rhodes, E.C.: A review of the concept of the heart rate deflection point. Sports Med. **30**(1), 31–46 (2000)
3. Brickley, G., Doust, J., Williams, C.: Physiological responses during exercise to exhaustion at critical power. Eur. J. Appl. Physiol. **88**(1–2), 146–151 (2002)
4. Brooke, J., Hamley, E.: The heart-rate–physical work curve analysis for the prediction of exhausting work ability. Med. Sci. Sports **4**(1), 23–26 (1972)
5. Brooke, J., Hamley, E., Thomason, H.: Relationship of heart rate to physical work. J. Physiol. **197**(1), 61P (1968)
6. Clingeleffer, A., Mc Naughton, L.R., Davoren, B.: The use of critical power as a determinant for establishing the onset of blood lactate accumulation. Eur. J. Appl. Physiol. Occup. Physiol. **68**(2), 182–187 (1994)
7. Ebert, T.R., Martin, D.T., McDonald, W., Victor, J., Plummer, J., Withers, R.T.: Power output during women's World Cup road cycle racing. J. Appl. Physiol. **95**, 8 (2005)
8. Ebert, T.R., Martin, D.T., Stephens, B., Withers, R.T.: Power output during a professional men's road-cycling tour. Int. J. Sports Physiol. Perform. **1**, 12 (2006)
9. Hill, A.V.: Muscular Movement In Man: The Factors Governing Speed and Recovery from Fatigue. McGraw-Hill, New York (1927)
10. Housh, D.J., Housh, T.J., Bauge, S.M.: The accuracy of the critical power test for predicting time to exhaustion during cycle ergometry. Ergonomics **32**(8), 997–1004 (1989)
11. Karsten, B., Jobson, S.A., Hopker, J., Stevens, L., Beedie, C.: Validity and reliability of critical power field testing. Eur. J. Appl. Physiol. **115**(1), 197–204 (2015)
12. Monod, H., Scherrer, J.: The work capacity of a synergic muscular group. Ergonomics **8**(3), 329–338 (1965)

13. Moritani, T., Nagata, A., Devries, H.A., Muro, M.: Critical power as measure of physical work capacity and anaerobic threshold. Ergonomics **24**(5), 339–350 (1981)
14. Quod, M., Martin, D., Martin, J., Laursen, P.: The power profile predicts road cycling MMP. Int. J. Sports Med. **31**(06), 397–401 (2010)
15. Rasmussen, C.E.: Gaussian processes in machine learning. In: Summer School on Machine Learning, pp. 63–71. Springer, Berlin (2003)
16. Vogt, S., Schumacher, Y., Roecker, K., Dickhuth, H.H., Schoberer, U., Schmid, A., Heinrich, L.: Power output during the tour de France. Int. J. Sports Med. **28**(9), 756–761 (2007)

Automatic Load Control
in Endurance Training

Katrin Hoffmann[(✉)]

Institut für Sportwissenschaft, Technische Universität Darmstadt,
Magdalenenstr. 27, 64289 Darmstadt, Germany
hoffmann@sport.tu-darmstadt.de

Abstract. Modeling and predicting load courses and HR responses enables
individually optimal training control. In HR controlled endurance training, load
is expected to gradually decrease to keep HR levels constant due to cardiac drift.
This paper analyzes if gender, time under load or progress of training influences
characteristics of load controlled by HR in continuous exercise during a long-
term training intervention. Nine healthy adults performed a twelve-week training
intervention on a bike ergometer. During the Intensive Continuous Method, load
was automatically adjusted (ALC) to keep individual HR in the range of 75%
$HR_{max} \pm 5$ bpm.

Load was reduced due to exceeding HR responses in all participants. Additionally, load increases were found in the first 5 and in the last 5 min of ALC.
A weak influence of gender on load increases was found. No further influence of
training, gender or time after onset of exercise was found. HR responses,
characteristics of cardiac drift, and corresponding load adjustments were highly
varying in individual participants. The findings should be integrated in HR
models to improve HR control and prediction.

Keywords: Modelling · Load courses · Cardiac drift · Individual HR response

1 Introduction

In the physical training process, it is essential to evoke individually optimal strain in the
human body to evoke responses corresponding to the training goals. Especially in
endurance training, heart rate (HR in beats per minute, bpm) is often used for pre-
scribing exercise intensity representing whole-body strain (Jeukendrup and Van Diemen 1998). HR controlled endurance training aims to apply load that is expected to
evoke individual optimal HR responses ($HR_{training}$) corresponding to predefined
training goals. Additionally, the load is adjusted throughout the training session to keep
these responses within a predefined training range.

Computer science in sports aims to provide a training control without overstraining
nor under challenging the trainee by modeling and predicting individual HR responses
and load courses. However, the high individuality of HR responses complicates this
optimal training control (Hoffmann et al. 2016).

One particular phenomena is the cardiac drift. This continuous increase in HR and
decrease in stroke volume during prolonged submaximal training is probably caused by

© Springer Nature Switzerland AG 2020
M. Lames et al. (Eds.): IACSS 2019, AISC 1028, pp. 132–139, 2020.
https://doi.org/10.1007/978-3-030-35048-2_16

hypovolemia and hyperthermia (Coyle and González-Alonso 2001). This effect is particular evident in long-term training sessions (Dawson et al. 2005, Jeukendrup and Van Diemen 1998) but was also detected in short training session lasting up to 30 min (Wingo et al. 2005). The underlying mechanisms causing cardiac drift are still controversial (Wingo et al. 2005).

Although a variety of possible HR models are currently available (Ludwig et al. 2018), the individuality of HR responses is up to date not sufficiently represented in these models. In particular, Cardiac Drift was integrated in only five of 25 analyzed models (Ludwig et al. 2018). Furthermore, most of these models only concentrate on HR responses. The influence of load adjustments during a training session in HR controlled training is often neglected. However, since HR and load are strongly correlated, especially the load course is important for training control in HR controlled endurance training. Regarding to literature, load is expected to be gradually decreased to keep HR levels constant (Wingo et al. 2005). This effect is particularly evident in the last part of exercise.

Therefore, this study investigated HR responses and load courses in HR controlled continuous exercise training during a long-term training intervention. In particular, the influence of gender, time under load or progress of training on these courses was evaluated. Furthermore, individual variances of the participants were analyzed.

2   Materials and Methods

The study presented here was approved by the Ethics Committee of the Technische Universität Darmstadt in 2016.

2.1   Participants and Apparatus

Nine healthy adults volunteered to participate in the study after having signed informed consent. All participants were non-smokers. No significant weight changes were measured during the training intervention. Participants' characteristics are displayed in Table 1.

All tests were performed using a cycle ergometer with a flywheel (Ergo Fit Ergometer 4000Med, Pirmasens, Germany). Power was controlled by the resistance at the flywheel and measured in Watts by the ergometer. HR data was assessed with a Polar chest belt (T31) and measured beat to beat by the ergometer. Data recording started at the beginning of the training protocol. Respiratory parameters were recorded using the spiroergometry device K5 (COSMED, Rome, Italy) during the testing procedures using a mixing chamber. First anaerobic threshold (ANT1) and second anaerobic threshold (ANT2) were automatically calculated from the respiratory parameters using OMNIA Software (COSMED, Rome, Italy).

Table 1. Demographic and anthropometric data of the participants

	Sex	Age [years]	Height [m]	Weight [kg]	BMI	Activity time per week [h]	Dietary habits
Participant 1	Male	24	1.78	82.3	23,1	>6	–
Participant 2	Male	28	1.83	96.1	26,3	<1.5	–
Participant 3	Male	34	1.90	78.1	20,6	<1.5	–
Participant 4	Male	25	1.68	76.5	22,8	<1.5	–
Participant 5	Female	24	1.65	87.2	26,4	>6	–
Participant 6	Female	22	1.70	69.0	20,3	4.5–6.0	–
Participant 7	Female	30	1.58	59.3	18,8	>6	–
Participant 8	Female	24	1.72	59.9	17,4	1.5–3.0	Vegetarian
Participant 9	Female	26	1.80	85.7	23,8	3.0–4.5	Pescetarian
Total *Mean*		26.3	1.73	77.1	22.2		
Total *SD*		3.74	0.09	12.5	3.1		

2.2 Protocol

All data was obtained during a twelve-week endurance training intervention on a bike ergometer. This duration was chosen as adaptations to the training can be reliably observed after this training period (Blank 2007). Prior to and after completion of the intervention, the participants performed an all-out exhaustion test to estimate the individual maximal HR (HR_{max}), the maximal Oxygen Uptake and the individual anaerobic thresholds (ANT1 and ANT2) of the participants. Additionally, two subtests were performed in week 4 and 8 to adapt the training intensity to the training status of the participants during the training process.

The protocol of the exhaustion test started with a resting period. Therefore, the participants sat still on the ergometer. After 3 min of rest, the participants started pedaling for 2 min at 25 W, followed by 3 min at 50 W. After this warm-up period, the load at the ergometer was gradually increased by 50 W every 3 min until exhaustion. In the subtests, the warm-up period of the exhaustion tests was repeated. Subsequently, the participants had to pass an exercise period of three increasing load levels for 3 min each. The load for these load levels was calculated to induce responses corresponding to the individual's anaerobic thresholds. Therefore, the first load was calculated to evoke responses below ANT1, the second load was calculated to evoke responses between ANT1 and ANT2 and the third load was calculated to evoke responses above ANT2. After this 9 min exercise period, a resting period of 5 min active recovery at 25 W was applied. Subsequently, another 9 min exercise period and 5 min recovery period were successively added to validate the results.

According to the guidelines of the WHO (WHO 2006) the training volume for the intervention was set to 25 min of intensive training three times a week following a 5 min warm-up phase according to the exhaustion test. Three different training methods were applied: the intensive continuous method (ICM), the extensive interval method (EIM) and the intensive interval method (IIM) (Hohmann et al. 2002). The load for each protocol was calculated to evoke $HR_{training}$ using the HR responses and corresponding load levels from the first exhaustion test and the subtests. The training protocols are displayed in Table 2 in detail.

Table 2. Protocols for the training intervention

	Intensive continuous method (ICM)	Extensive interval method (EIM)	Intensive interval method (IIM)
Intensity	75% HR_{max}	85% HR_{max}	95% HR_{max}
Load period	25 min	3:30 min	1:00 min
Recovery time between load intervals	0 min	1:30 min	1:30 min
Repetitions	1	5	10

All protocols were automatically applied at the ergometer. The participants were advised to keep the pedal rate (PR) constant at 80 revolutions per minute (RPM).

In ICM, the load that was expected to evoke 75% HR_{max} was set at the ergometer for 5 min. Thus, HR was allowed to slowly increase to the $HR_{training}$. Subsequently, the Automatic Load Control (ALC) was applied at the ergometer until the end of exercise. In the ALC, HR responses were compared to the predefined $HR_{training}$ range (75% $HR_{max} \pm 5$ bpm) every 60 s. In case the HR exceeded or fell below this range, load was automatically increased or reduced by 10 W.

2.3 Data Analysis

In this study, only data of the ICM training protocols were analyzed representing HR controlled endurance training. The individual HR of the participants is expected to stay rather constant due to the particular training protocol. Therefore, the adjustment of load corresponding to individual HR responses were analyzed.

In total, HR and load courses of 108 training sessions were analyzed. Three courses were excluded due to measuring errors. Data was analyzed 10 min after onset of load until the end of exercise. Thus, only HR and load courses during ALC were included in analysis.

MANOVA was performed to examine the influence of gender and week of training on number of load increases ($Load_{inc}$), number of load reductions ($Load_{red}$) and total number of load adjustments during the training sessions. Additionally, ANOVA with repeated measures was performed to investigate the influence of time under load on $Load_{inc}$ and $Load_{red}$. Therefore, Time under load was grouped together in 10–14 min after onset of exercise, 15–19 min after onset of exercise, 20–24 min after onset of exercise and 25–29 min after onset of exercise. All statistical analyses were performed with IBM SPSS Statistics 24.

3 Results

For all participants, the mean HR during ALC was slightly elevated compared to HR$_{training}$. ($M = 0.8$ BPM, $SD = 0.63$ BPM). The appearance of cardiac drift was recognizable during the training intervention in all participants. Therefore, load was reduced (Load$_{red}$) due to exceeding HR responses in all participants. Due to varying responses, the characteristics of corresponding load adjustments were also varying between the participants. This includes on the one hand the total number of Load$_{red}$, for individual participants, but also the number of Load$_{red}$ per training session. Participant 9 did not show a Load$_{red}$ in three training sessions caused by rather constant HR responses with minor variations within the expected training range. Nevertheless, an increase in HR was found (HR response 14 min after onset of exercise averaged over 30 s: 136.6 BPM, HR response 29 min after onset of exercise averaged over 30 s: 142.1 BPM). Additionally, the total number of 14 Load$_{red}$ in participant 9 was well below the group mean ($M = 33.8$, $SD = 11.05$).

In contrast to the expectations, a high number of Load$_{inc}$ was found in all participants throughout the training. In participant 9, even more Load$_{inc}$ than Load$_{red}$ were recorded. Averaged HR responses and number of load adjustments for all participants are displayed in Table 3.

Table 3. HR responses and number of load adjustments of each participant during ALC (10 min after onset until the end of exercise). Legend: Mean Load$_{inc}$/Load$_{red}$: Mean value of load increases/reductions during single training sessions; Total Load$_{inc}$/Load$_{red}$: Total amount of load increases/reduction during the training intervention (12 weeks).

	Mean HR [BPM]	SD HR [BPM]	HR$_{training}$ [BPM]	Mean Load$_{inc}$	SD Load$_{inc}$	Mean Load$_{red}$	SD Load$_{red}$	Total Load$_{inc}$	Total Load$_{red}$
Participant 1	145.0	4.0	144	2.1	1.24	2.3	0.62	18	27
Participant 2	156.1	4.7	156	2.1	1.31	2.8	1.49	24	33
Participant 3	141.9	4.6	140	2.1	1.49	3.8	1.71	16	46
Participant 4	149.4	4.6	149	2.0	1.36	2.6	1.92	22	31
Participant 5	131.7	3.9	131	1,8	1.47	3.3	1.44	15	39
Participant 6	150.8	5.4	150	1.6	1.22	3.9	1.03	32	43
Participant 7	141.2	5.1	140	1.2	1.19	3.9	0.84	21	47
Participant 8	144.1	4.3	143	1.3	1.00	2.4	1.31	20	24
Participant 9	136.8	4.4	137	2.2	1.04	1.2	1.38	29	14

A significant interaction term of training week and gender on number of Load$_{inc}$ was found ($F = 2.19$, $p < 0.05$, $\eta^2 = 0.23$). Particularly, gender was revealed as main effect with a very low effect size ($F = 4.47$, $p < 0.05$, $\eta^2 = 0.05$). No influence of gender and training week was found on either number of Load$_{red}$ ($F = 0.29$, $p > 0.05$) nor total number of adjustments ($F = 1.52$, $p > 0.05$).

The total number of adjustments during training showed significant differences between participants ($F = 2.78$, $p < 0.01$, $\eta^2 = 0.19$). Interestingly, no significant difference was found for the number of $Load_{inc}$ ($F = 1.07$, $p > 0.05$) but for the number of $Load_{red}$ ($F = 5.49$, $p < 0.01$, $\eta^2 = 0.31$). Bonferroni corrected pairwise comparison revealed highly significant differences of participant 9 ($M = 1.2$, $SD = 0.84$) to participant 3 ($M = 3.8$, $SD = 1.34$), participant 5 ($M = 3.3$, $SD = 1.71$), participant 6 ($M = 3.9$, $SD = 1.92$), and participant 7 ($M = 3.9$, $SD = 1.44$). Two prototypical HR and load courses are displayed in Figs. 1 and 2.

A significant difference of $Load_{inc}$ were found for the distinct time slots ($F = 49.43$; $p = .00$; $\eta^2 = .861$). Bonferroni corrected pairwise comparison revealed significant higher $Load_{inc}$ in the first 10–14 min after onset of exercise ($p < .01$). An elevated but not significantly different number of $Load_{inc}$ were also found in the last five minutes of ALC. No significant differences regarding the number of $Load_{red}$ at distinct time slopts were found. However, $Load_{red}$ was elevated between 15 and 19 min after onset of exercise. In contrast to the expectations, number of $Load_{red}$ was neither increasing throughout the training nor increased in the last part of the training session.

The number of load adjustments in particular time slots are displayed in Table 4.

Table 4. Number of load adjustments during ALC in distinct time slots. Note: ALC started 10 min after onset.

	10–14 min	15–19 min	20–24 min	25–29 min	Total
Load increases	132	15	18	28	193
Load reductions	69	99	66	72	306

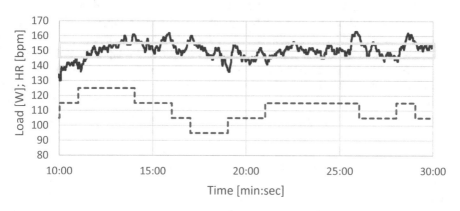

Fig. 1. Prototypical load, HR courses and HR training zones of a female participant during ALC. HR training range: 150 bpm ± 5 bpm, Training week 3. In total: 5 load increases and 5 load reductions throughout the training due to highly varying HR responses.

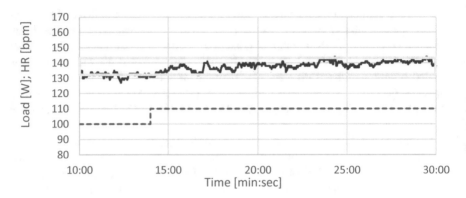

Fig. 2. Prototypical load, HR courses and HR training zones of a female participant during the ALC. HR training range: 137 bpm ± 5 bpm, Training week 3. In total: one load increase.

4   Discussions

As expected, the cardiac drift causing Load$_{red}$ was found in all participants. In the analyzed sample, no effect of gender or training week on Load$_{red}$ was found. Furthermore, Load$_{red}$ was significantly varying in individual participants due to varying HR responses. This indicates that the characteristics of cardiac drift are varying individually, independent of gender or training status. The varying results are possibly due to varying training status prior to the training intervention and the small sample size. Additionally, influences of varying weather conditions are possible. Due to a lack of air conditioning it was not possible to keep the temperature in the laboratory precisely constant throughout the training interventions. Furthermore, weather-sensitive participants occasionally felt uncomfortable due to fluctuating air pressure.

Similar to Load$_{red}$, a high amount of Load$_{inc}$ was also found throughout the training session. The Load$_{inc}$ in the first minutes of ALC was probably caused by the conservative load application in order to prevent overstraining. However, a successive increase of three or more Load$_{inc}$ was found in individual participants after onset of ALC. This behavior was not expected as the load was particularly calculated to evoke HR$_{training}$.

Load$_{inc}$ was also elevated in the last 5 min of training. In 13 analyzed data sets, the load was even elevated until the end of training. There is a tendency, that the number of Load$_{inc}$ is smaller in females than in males. However, due to the low effect size the results need to be validated in a larger sample. The occurrence of this high amount of Load$_{inc}$ is possibly due to the small tolerance for HR variances during the ALC. Therefore, load adjustments caused by HR variability are possible. This effect is confirmed by the high amount of load adjustments during ALC of participants with highly varying HR responses. However, the occurrence of Load$_{inc}$ contradicts current literature und should be analyzed in more detail in future research.

The presented findings are very important for modeling HR responses. In current HR models, cardiac drift is, if any, mostly integrated as constant. The findings indicate that no generalized statements can be made. The integration of cardiac drift in HR models has to include individual patterns. Especially, individual HR responses to the change of load might be a possibility to improve the integration. Furthermore, the results clearly demonstrated that the influence of cardiac drift on HR can be reduced and even briefly neutralized. This effect is especially important for the use of HR models in practice. Modeling load courses in HR controlled endurance training therefore requires the integration of cardiac drift even in short term training sessions. Individual and precise analysis of HR responses is necessary to improve HR models. Further research is needed addressing individual characteristics of cardiac drift and corresponding load courses.

5 Conclusions

In the analyzed sample, adjustments enabling load control corresponding to HR responses were found in all participants. Load reductions caused by cardiac drift as well as load increased were found throughout the training intervention independent of training, gender or time under load in the presented sample. Only a weak influence of gender on load increases was found. Modeling load courses providing individual endurance training corresponding to predefined HR training zone requires the integration of the high individuality of HR responses.

References

Blank, M.: Dimensionen und Determinanten der Trainierbarkeit Konditioneller Fähigkeiten. Czwalina, Hamburg (2007)

Coyle, E.F., Gonzalez-Alonso, J.: Cardiovascular drift during prolonged exercise: new perspectives. Exerc. Sport Sci. Rev. 29(2), 88–92 (2001)

Dawson, E.A., Shave, R., George, K., Whyte, G., Ball, D., Gaze, D., Collinson, P.: Cardiac drift during prolonged exercise with echocardiographic evidence of reduced diastolic function of the heart. Eur. J. Appl. Physiol. 94(3), 305–309 (2005)

Hohmann, A., Lames, M., Letzelter, M.: Einführung in die Trainingswissenschaft. Limpert Verlag, Wiebelsheim (2002)

Hoffmann, K., Wiemeyer, J., Hardy, S.: Prediction and control of the individual Heart Rate response in Exergames. In: Chung, P., Soltoggio, A., Dawson, C.W., Meng, Q., Pain, M. (eds.) Proceedings of the 10th International Symposium on Computer Science in Sports (ISCSS). AISC, vol. 392, pp. 171–178. Springer, Cham (2016). https://doi.org/10.1007/978-3-319-24560-7_22

Jeukendrup, A., Diemen, A.V.: Heart rate monitoring during training and competition in cyclists. J. Sports Sci. 16(sup1), 91–99 (1998)

Loellgen, H., Graham, T., Sjogaard, G.: Muscle metabolites, force, and perceived exertion bicycling at varying pedal rates. Med. Sci. Sports Exerc. 12, 345–351 (1980)

Ludwig, M., Hoffmann, K., Endler, S., Asteroth, A., Wiemeyer, J.: Measurement prediction and control of individual heart rate responses to exercise—basics and options for wearable devices. Front. Physiol. 9, 778 (2018)

Wingo, J., LaFrenz, A., Ganio, M., Edwards, G., Cureton, K.: Cardiovascular drift is related to reduced maximal oxygen uptake during heat stress. Med. Sci. Sports Exerc. 37(2), 248–255 (2005)

World Health Organisation [WHO]: Constitution of the WHO. Basic Documents 45 (Supplement, October 2006), pp. 1–18 (2006)

Other Application Fields

Blood Flow Under Mechanical Stimulations

Timur Gamilov[1,2] and Sergey Simakov[1,2(✉)]

[1] Sechenov University, 19s1, Bol'shaya Pirogovskaya Ulitsa, Moscow 119146, Russia
gamilov@crec.mipt.ru
[2] Moscow Institute of Physics and Technology, 9, Institutsky per.,
Dolgoprudny 141701, Russia
simakov.ss@mipt.ru
https://www.sechenov.ru/
https://www.mipt.ru/

Abstract. We propose a one-dimensional blood flow model taking into account muscle pump, external contraction and autoregulation. This model is used to study two effects: blood flow during running and the impact of enhanced external counterpulsation on the coronary blood flow on the basis of patient-specific data. On the basis of mathematical modelling we observe optimal stride frequency, which maximizes venous return.

Keywords: Coronary blood flow · Muscle pump · Enhanced external counterpulsation · Stride frequency

1 Introduction

Cardiovascular system is a major limiting factor in high performance sport. The blood flow delivers nutrients (such as O_2 or glucose) to the muscles and remove metabolic wastes (CO_2) [5]. Intensive periodic physical activity is associated with increased heart outflow. Periodic muscle contractions result in additional external pressure applied to the vessel's walls, which may lead to either negative or positive effect. A similar effect can be produced by enhanced external counterpulsation (EECP). EECP involves surrounding patient's legs and lower abdomen with inflatable cuffs that are pressurized and depressurized during diastole [8]. EECP impulses are synchronized with the heart beats using the electrocardiogram (ECG) and blood pressure monitors. This allows to direct additional blood stored in the lower extremities towards the heart therefore improve blood supply of the heart tissues. EECP improves cardiac performance, stimulate angiogenesis, reactive hyperemia and flow-mediated dilation in peripheral arteries. It is also used as a method of recovery from high-intensity interval training [2]. Effectiveness of this method in sport is still discussed [11].

In this work we follow the approach [7,10] of global dynamical 1D network hemodynamics simulation as a flow of viscous incompressible fluid through the

© Springer Nature Switzerland AG 2020
M. Lames et al. (Eds.): IACSS 2019, AISC 1028, pp. 143–150, 2020.
https://doi.org/10.1007/978-3-030-35048-2_17

network of elastic tubes. We consider both arterial and venous parts of the systemic circulation. We use computational domain extracted from physiologically correct data set [9]. The network structure of the coronary part is reconstructed from patient-specific data. Arterial autoregulation and venous valve functioning for lower extremities model are included following [3,10]. Myocardial action in coronary part simulated by applying external pressure and increased resistance of the appropriate vessels. EECP regimes are implemented similar to the [8]. The cuffs pressure model is quite similar to the muscles contraction model presented in [10]. We study the effects of vessel wall elasticity and autoregulation on the coronary circulation during EECP.

We also use developed model to study the effect of muscle pump on the blood flow in lower extremities. Skeletal-muscle pump effect is introduced as an external time-periodical pressure function applied to a group of the veins. Period of this function is associated with the two strides period during running. On the basis of mathematical modelling we observe optimal stride frequency, which maximizes the venous return.

2   Methods

2.1   Blood Flow Model

In this work we follow the approach [10] of global dynamical 1D network hemodynamics simulation as a flow of viscous incompressible fluid through the network of elastic tubes.

$$\partial A_k/\partial t + \partial \left(A_k u_k \right)/\partial x = 0, \tag{1}$$

$$\partial u_k/\partial t + \partial \left(u_k^2/2 + p_k/\rho \right)/\partial x = f_{fr} \left(A_k, u_k \right), \tag{2}$$

where k is an index of the vessel; t is time; x is distance along the vessel counted from the vessel's junction point; ρ is blood density (constant); $A_k \left(t, x \right)$ is vessels's cross-section area; p_k is blood pressure; $u_k \left(t, x \right)$ is linear velocity averaged over the cross-section; f_{tr} is a friction force.

Elastic properties of the vessel wall material are described by the wall-state equation providing response to the transmural pressure (the difference between blood pressure and pressure in the tissues surrounding the vessel)

$$p_k \left(A_k \right) - p_{*k} = \rho c_k^2 f \left(A_k \right), \tag{3}$$

where $f \left(A_k \right)$ is an S-like function [10], p_{*k} is pressure in the tissues surrounding the vessel, c_k is small disturbances propagation velocity of the wall material. Term p_{*k} is used to simulate pressure from the cuff or muscles.

Extended review of similar 1D models can be found in [1].

2.2   Autoregulation

Vessels are capable of changing their elastic properties in response to change of the averaged blood flow parameters. This effect is usually referred to as autoregulation [6]. The increase in mean pressure results in the vascular smooth muscle contraction which results in higher pulse wave velocity. The same is valid for the mean pressure decrease resulting in lower pulse wave velocity.

The model of the arterial autoregulation used in this work is described also in [10]. We assume that vessel tend to keep its cross-section constant by changing its stiffness. It can be described as dependence of parameter c_k in (3) from average pressure $\bar{p}_k$. We update the value of c_k every averaging period. New value is defined by

$$\frac{c_{k,new}}{c_{k,old}} = \sqrt{\frac{\bar{p}_{k,new}}{\bar{p}_{k,old}}}, \tag{4}$$

where $\bar{p}_{k,new} = \dfrac{\int_{T_2}^{T_3} \int_0^{l_k} p(x,t)dxdt}{(T_3 - T_2)l_k}$; $\bar{p}_{k,old} = \dfrac{\int_{T_1}^{T_2} \int_0^{l_k} p(x,t)dxdt}{(T_2 - T_1)l_k}$; l_k is a length of k-th vessel; T_1, T_2, T_3, T_4 are the moments when cardiac cycle starts.

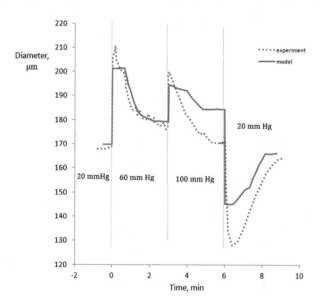

Fig. 1. Effect of pressure changes on diameter of cannulated rat artery (experimental data [12]). Initial pressure was set to 20 mmHg, from this baseline steps were applied to 60 mmHg and to 100 mmHg, and back to 20 mmHg. Averaging period of autoregulation is set to 50 s.

c_k changes gradually over averaging period:

$$c_k = c_{k,old} + \gamma \frac{t - T_3}{T_4 - T_3}(c_{k,new} - c_{k,old}), \tag{5}$$

where $0 \leq \gamma \leq 1$ is the parameter reflecting the autoregulation intensity. We associate the value $\gamma = 1$ with the normal case and $\gamma < 1$ with autoregulation that is impaired due to some reasons (endothelial dysfunction, vasodilator drugs). $\gamma = 0$ means that there is no autoregulation. Figure 1 shows simulation of autoregulation effect on a single vessel.

2.3   Mechanical Stimulations Model

The results of anatomically correct data processing from [9] presented in [3] are used in this work as basic 1D structure of systemic circulation. Patient specific data are processed by an algorithm [4] to obtain the structure of coronary arteries.

A three-step graded-sequential compression procedure described in [8] was used in all simulations. Three pressure cuffs sequentially apply pressure to calves, thighs and lower abdomen as schematically presented at Fig. 2. In this work cuff pressure is simulated by p_{*k} in (3). The pressure in each cuff instantly rises to its maximum value P_{ext} at the moment of time T_s and drops to zero at T_f as shown at Fig. 3. Parameters' values for each region of cuffs are specified in the Table 1.

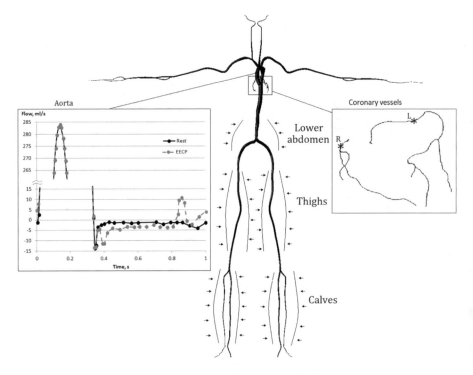

Fig. 2. Vessels affected by cuffs pressure. Effect of EECP on aortic blood flow: retrograde blood flow at the beginning of diastole (around 0.4 s) and antegrade blood flow at the end of diastole (around 0.8–1.0 s). L: left coronary artery, R: right coronary artery.

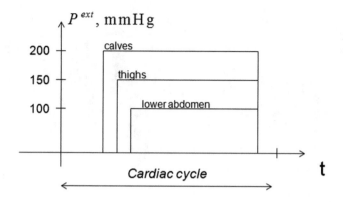

Fig. 3. Cuffs pressure during the heart cycle (see Table 1).

Table 1. EECP parameters for each zone. Notations are presented on Fig. 3

	Cuffs pressure	Timing (see [8])	
	P_{ext}, mm hg	T_s, s	T_f, s
Calves	200	0.24	0.8
Thighs	150	0.25	0.8
Lower abdomen	100	0.26	0.8

3   Results

3.1   EECP Simulations

Two series of simulations were performed. The duration of EECP treatment in each simulation is one hour. Average blood flow and average blood pressure are studied in different parts of coronary network. Averaging period for autoregulatory response equals to 1 cardiac cycle.

First series contains simulations for vessels with different elasticity described by parameter c in (3). Higher values of c correspond to stiffer vessels which can be caused by different systemic diseases (e.g. atherosclerosis, calcinosis), aging, prolonged alcohol consumption, et al. Lower values of c correspond to more elastic vessels. It can be caused by endurance sports (running). We study average pressure and flow in coronary artery in the range of -30% decrease up to 30% increase in elasticity. Figure 4 shows that EECP procedure is less effective (in terms of the coronary blood flow) for the patient with more elastic vessels. This may decrease the effect of cardiovascular workout during EECP therapy for certain groups of athletes, e.g. long distance runners (long distance runners tend to have lower arterial stiffness [10]).

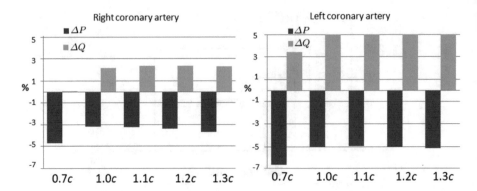

Fig. 4. Change in average pressure (ΔP) and average flow (ΔQ) during EECP procedure. c – reference values for right and left coronary arteries. LCA: $P_{ave} = 74$ mmHg, $Q_{ave} = 33$ ml/min, RCA: $P_{ave} = 72$ mmHg, $Q_{ave} = 8$ ml/min.

Second series studies the impact of autoregulation on the changes in blood flow during EECP. Three cases were simulated: normal autoregulation ($\gamma = 1$), restrained autoregulation ($\gamma = 0.5$) and absence of autoregulation ($\gamma = 0$). The latter two cases may be associated with vasodilator or vasoconstrictor drugs administration or endothelial dysfunction. Figure 5 represents average pressure and flow difference in these three cases. We can see clearly that autoregulation results in negative response to EECP action. Thus, its suppression may be recommended to achieve greater blood supply of coronary vessels. Some limitations should be considered in this case due to simultaneous pressure increase in aorta.

3.2   Muscle Pump Simulations

We use model to study effects of skeletal-muscle pumping on the blood flow in lower extremities [10]. Skeletal-muscle pump effect is introduced as an external time-periodical pressure function applied to a group of the veins. Period of this function is associated with the two strides period during running. Computational study reveals explicit optimal stride frequency providing maximum blood flow through the lower extremities. We estimate this optimal frequency for a variety of heights (Fig. 6A, B, C, D). The value of blood flow increase is not substantial, but the value of optimal frequency can be estimated near the maximum. From Fig. 6 one can observe quite good agreement between simulated and actual optimal stride frequencies in the wide range of heights.

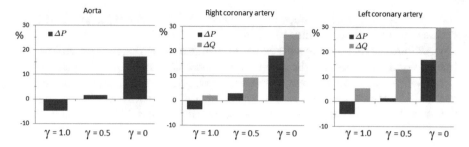

Fig. 5. Change in average pressure (ΔP) and average flow (ΔQ) during EECP procedure for different autoregulation function. $\gamma = 1$ – normal autoregulation; $\gamma = 0.5$ –
restrained autoregulation; $\gamma = 0$ – absence of autoregulation. Aorta: $P_{ave} = 90$ mmHg,
LCA: $P_{ave} = 74$ mmHg, $Q_{ave} = 33$ ml/min, RCA: $P_{ave} = 72$ mmHg, $Q_{ave} = 8$ ml/min.

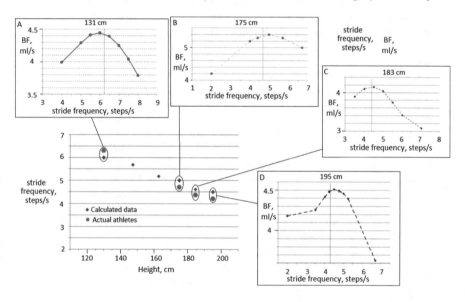

Fig. 6. Stride frequencies of trained athletes (circles) and calculated optimal frequencies (diamonds) for different heights. A, B, C, D: blood flow (BF) as a function of
stride frequency for four different heights. Vertical lines on A, B, C, D represent actual
frequency of real athletes with corresponding heights.

4   Conclusion

Results show that EECP therapy can have different effect on different groups of
athletes. Athletes with more elastic vessels may not experience any significant
increase in blood supply of the heart. Simulations for the case of absent autoregulation demonstrate significant increase in coronary blood flow. It shows that
administration of vasodilator drugs can have severe effect on ECCP procedure.
We conclude that EECP therapy should be adjusted for each athlete. Vasodila-

tor drugs can be used to improve the effect of EECP therapy, but additional studies are needed to minimize the risk.

Computational study reveals explicit optimal stride frequency providing maximum blood flow through the lower extremities. Optimal stride frequency computed by our method strongly correlates with observations. Deviation between calculated optimal frequencies and actual stride frequencies of elite runners do not exceed 10%, although the deviation observed for non-trained person is larger.

References

1. Bessonov, T.N., Sequeira, A., Simakov, S., Vassilevskii, Y., Volpert, V.: Methods of blood flow modelling. Math. Mod. Nat. Phenom. **11**(1), 1–25 (2016)
2. Bozorgi, A., Mehrabi Nasab, E., Sardari, A., Nejatian, M., Nasirpour, S., Sadeghi, S.: Effect of enhanced external counterpulsation (EECP) on exercise time duration and functional capacity in patients with refractory angina pectoris. J. Tehran Heart Cent. **9**(1), 33–37 (2014)
3. Gamilov, T., Ivanov, Y., Kopylov, P., Simakov, S., Vassilevski, Y.: Patient specific haemodynamic modeling after occlusion treatment in leg. Math. Model. Nat. Phenom. **9**(6), 85–97 (2014). https://doi.org/10.1051/mmnp/20149607
4. Gamilov, T.M., Kopylov, P.Y., Pryamonosov, R.A., Simakov, S.S.: Virtual fractional flow reserve assesment in patient-specific coronary networks by 1D hemodynamic model (FFR). Rus. J. Num. Anal. Math. Mod. **5**, 269–276 (2015)
5. Golov, A.V., Simakov, S.S.: Mathematical model of respiratory regulation during hypoxia and hypercapnia. Comp. Res. Mod. **9**(2), 297–310 (2017)
6. Johnson, P.C.: Autoregulation of blood flow. Circ. Res. **59**, 482–495 (1986)
7. Kholodov, A.S.: Some dynamical models of external breathing and blood circulation regarding to their interaction and substances transfer. In: Belotsirkovsky, O.M., Kholodov, A.S. (eds.) Computational Models and Medicine Progress, pp. 127–163. Science, Moscow (2001)
8. Ozawa, E.T., Bottom, K.E., Xiao, X., Kamm, R.D.: Numerical simulation of enhanced external counterpulsation. Ann. Biomed. Eng. **29**, 284–297 (2001)
9. Plasticboy Pictures CC (2009). http://www.plasticboy.co.uk/store/
10. Simakov, S.S., Gamilov, T.M., Soe, Y.N.: Computational study of blood flow in lower extremities under intense physical load. Russ. J. Numer. Anal. Math. Model. **28**(5), 485–504 (2013)
11. Valenzuela, P.L., Montalvo, Z., Torrontegi, E., Sánchez-Martínez, G., Lucia, A., De la Villa, P.: Enhanced external counterpulsation and recovery from a plyometric exercise bout. Clin. J. Sport Med. (2018). https://doi.org/10.1097/JSM.0000000000000620
12. VanBavel, E., van der Meulen, E.T., Spaan, J.A.: Role of Rho-associated protein kinase in tone and calcium sensitivity of cannulated rat mesenteric small arteries. Exp. Physiol. **86**(5), 585–592 (2001)

Polygenic Modeling of Muscle Fibers Composition

Oleg Borisov[1(✉)], Carlo Maj[1], Nikolay Kulemin[2],
Ekaterina Semenova[2], Peter Krawitz[1], Ildus Ahmetov[2,3],
and Edward Generozov[2]

[1] Institute for Genomic Statistics and Bioinformatics, University Hospital Bonn,
Sigmund-Freud-Straße 25, 53127 Bonn, Germany
olegbor@uni-bonn.de
[2] Federal Research and Clinical Center of Physical-Chemical Medicine
of Federal Medical Biological Agency, 1A Malaya Pirogovskaya,
119992 Moscow, Russia
[3] Kazan State Medical University, 49 Butlerov Street, 420012 Kazan, Russia

Abstract. The present study investigated the genetic architecture of muscle
fibers composition by means of the genome-wide association study and polygenic score modeling. Hundred thousands of single genetic variants and aggregated signal from multiple genetic variants were tested for an association with a
proportion of the type I muscle fibers. We found several suggestively associated
genetic variants (p-value < 0.00001) that can be potentially replicated with a
larger cohort. The polygenic scores for 165 individuals using 49,105 genetic
variants identified a significant association between the polygenic component and
muscle fibers ratio (linear regression p-value = 0.00012). The present work
provides new insights into the complex genetic structure of the muscle fibers.

Keywords: Muscle fibers composition · Genome-wide association study ·
Polygenic scores modeling

1 Introduction

Recent technological advances in genetics have allowed to perform genome-wide
association studies and identify genetics markers associated with different human traits
(Balding 2006). Multifactorial traits, such as muscle fibers composition, are usually
connected to multiple loci, each explaining a small part of heritability (Yang et al.
2011). To aggregate the signal from those loci into one value per individual, the
method of polygenic scoring is widely used (Dudbridge 2013). Several genetic models
for the muscle fibers and athletic performance are present in the literature (Ahmetov
et al. 2012; Borisov et al. 2018). The present study aimed at investigating the association between hundreds of thousands of the single genetic variants and the proportion
of the type I muscle fibers (phenotype). Polygenic scores were constructed as an effect
size weighted combination of multiple genetic markers and tested for the association
with the phenotype. The best-fitting model of polygenic scores was selected and the
proportion of explained phenotypic variance was assessed.

© Springer Nature Switzerland AG 2020
M. Lames et al. (Eds.): IACSS 2019, AISC 1028, pp. 151–158, 2020.
https://doi.org/10.1007/978-3-030-35048-2_18

2   Materials and Method

The sample consisted of 171 individuals (115 males and 56 females). For each sample, the muscle biopsy with the subsequent immunohistochemical staining was performed to assess the proportion of muscle fibers (type I and type II). As a phenotype, we selected the proportion of type I fibers. These values were normally distributed (Shapiro-Wilk normality test, p = 0.59). There was no significant difference between the distribution of the type I fibers proportion in males comparing to females (Welch Two Sample t-test, p = 0.15). We standardized these values to mean = 0 and standard deviation = 1. The distribution of the phenotype is given in Fig. 1. The values above zero indicate the predominance of type I fibers while the values below zero indicate the predominance of type II fibers.

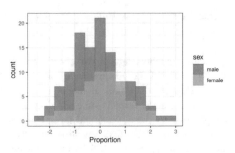

Fig. 1. Histogram of the phenotype distribution in both sexes. X-axis – standardized proportion of type 1 muscle fibers, Y-axis – number of samples.

2.1   Genotyping

For all 171 samples, the high-throughput genotyping using the BeadChip genotyping array (960,000 genetic markers) was performed. Since the polygenic score is known to be influenced by population stratification (Curtis 2018), we performed principal component analysis (PCA) to control for population substructure (see Fig. 2).

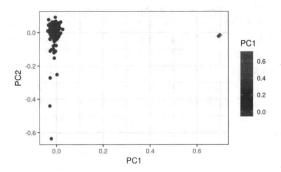

Fig. 2. PCA results. X-axis – Principal component 1, Y-axis – Principal component 2.

The first principal component of 2 samples and the second principal component of 4 samples deviated more than 3 standard deviations from the mean, so these samples were excluded.

We removed all variants with minor allele frequency (MAF) lower than 0.05. All variants with missing call rates exceeding 0.1 were filtered out. The variants with Hardy-Weinberg equilibrium exact test p-value below 1e−10 were also filtered out. We ended up with 609,028 variants and 165 samples.

2.2 Genome-Wide Association Study

We started from conducting the genome-wide association study (GWAS). We tested each variant against the phenotype using the linear regression. The results of the GWAS were presented as summary statistics containing beta coefficients and regression p-values. The GWAS was followed by the multiple comparison correction using the false discovery rate (FDR) method. The presence of the genetic signal was assessed by means of the quantile-quantile (Q-Q) probability plot.

2.3 Polygenic Scores Modeling

The sample of 165 people was divided into two groups - a training sample (110 samples, 2/3 of the total sample) and a test sample (55 samples, 1/3 of the total sample). Beta coefficients and p-values for each of the genetic variants were calculated for the training sample from the linear regression. The polygenic model for each individual in the test sample was constructed as a weighted sum of the single genetic variants effects divided by the total number of variants. The effect of each variant was calculated as a product of the beta coefficient of the training sample summary statistics and the number of minor alleles in an individual of the test sample (0, 1 or 2). Polygenic scores were calculated for the test sample after clumping to filter out linked genetic variants. We calculated the scores at 100 p-value thresholds from $p <= 5e−05$ with a logarithmic step to the full model including all variants at $p <= 1$. In total, we performed 1,000 random sampling iterations, and the polygenic scores for each individual were averaged. Among 100 models, we selected the best fitting one based on the highest R^2 from the linear regression.

2.4 Software

For the preprocessing step and quality control we used PLINK 1.90 (Chang et al. 2015). To calculate the polygenic scores, we used PRSice-2 (Euesden et al. 2015). For data handing and plotting, we used GNU bash, version 4.2.46, R version 3.4.4, and the "qqman" library (Turner 2018). The computing was performed on the high-performance computing cluster with 18 computational nodes of 64–256 GB RAM.

3   Results

3.1   Genome-Wide Association Study

The GWAS summary statistics is illustrated as a Manhattan (scatter) plot. Each dot on the plot represents a single genetic variant that was tested. On Y-axis of the plot, the negative logarithm of the association p-value is given, on X-axis – 22 chromosomes and X (23rd) chromosome. The blue horizontal line illustrates the significance level 1e−5. The variants with the significance below this level were considered as suggestively associated with the phenotype. The Manhattan plot is given in Fig. 3.

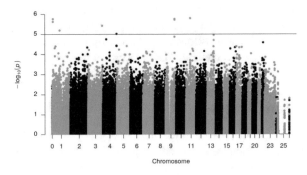

Fig. 3. Manhattan plot of GWAS results. X-axis – chromosomes, Y-axis – negative logarithm of p-value

Suggestively associated variants are given the Table 1.

Table 1. Suggestively associated genetic variants (CHR - chromosome, A1 – risk allele, q-value – adjusted p-value).

CHR	Genetic variant	bp	A1	Beta	p-value	q-value
11	rs504661	55312683	G	0.56	0.0000016	0.29
1	rs2003046	11032827	A	−0.66	0.0000017	0.29
9	rs7028883	120717586	A	0.69	0.0000017	0.29
9	rs10115978	120728632	A	0.7	0.0000019	0.29
1	rs11121667	11038476	A	−0.64	0.0000023	0.29
3	rs12632821	188586447	A	0.51	0.0000037	0.38
1	rs12405027	101927038	C	0.91	0.0000063	0.56
4	rs13102235	186373316	G	−0.5	0.0000094	0.73

After multiple comparison correction (FDR) the lowest q-value (adjusted p-value) was 0.29. However, we were observing some inflation at the Q-Q plot (deviation of the observed p-values from the expected p-values) that can witness the presence of the polygenic signal (see Fig. 4).

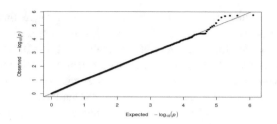

Fig. 4. Quantile-quantile plot of the association results. X-axis – expected negative logarithm of p-values, Y-axis – observed values

3.2   Polygenic Scores Modeling

Each polygenic score model at different thresholds included a different number of variants, the summary of them is given in Table 2.

Table 2. Number of variants included in the polygenic score at several p-value thresholds

Before clumping		After clumping	
Threshold	N of variants	Threshold	N of variant
0.000123	75	0.000123	47
0.000910	587	0.000910	316
0.006730	4282	0.006730	1990
0.135000	93060	0.135000	23675
1.000000	609028	1.000000	78019

The distribution of polygenic scores at these thresholds are shown in Fig. 5.

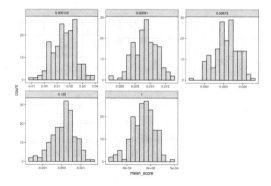

Fig. 5. Histograms of polygenic scores. X-axis – averaged polygenic scores, Y-axis – number of samples. P-value thresholds are given in the grey header of each panel.

We assessed the distributions of scores at different p-value threshold using the Shapiro-Wilk normality test. Among 100 thresholds, 47 scores distribution deviated from the normal distribution (Shapiro-Wilk normality test p < 0.05). After FDR correction the lowest Shapiro-Wilk p-value was greater than 0.1 (none stayed significant). The nominally significant deviation from the normal distribution correlated with the higher variance explained (p < 2.2e−16). Among 100 models, the best-fitting one was found at the p-value threshold 0.0742 which included 49,105 genetic variants. The distribution of p-values and R^2 of all 100 models is presented in Fig. 6.

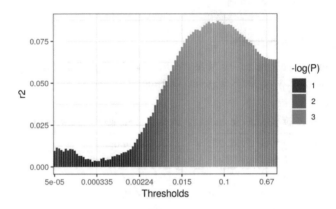

Fig. 6. Barplot illustrating the model R^2 (Y-axis) at different p-value threshold (X-axis)

Finally, the linear regression between the phenotypic values and the scores produced significant results (p = 0.00012, R^2 = 0.087). We found that the polygenic scores within the best-fitting model were significantly associated with the type I muscle fibers proportion. The regression results are presented in Fig. 7.

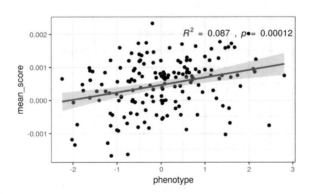

Fig. 7. Linear regression between the scores (Y-axis) and phenotypes (X-axis).

4   Discussion

This work has investigated the genetic structure of the muscle fibers composition using the type I fibers proportion as a phenotype. We performed the genome-wide association study followed by the polygenic modeling to combine the multiple genetic effect into a single score. Our genome-wide association study revealed 8 suggestive single nucleotide variants that reached the threshold $p < 1e-5$. Of those, the SNP rs12632821 (located in the LPP gene) can be the most relevant to muscle fibre function, given its role in the cytoskeletal signaling. We did not find any significantly associated genetic variant after the multiple comparison correction. However, it can be explained by a relatively small sample size. Therefore, we tried to combine the signal from multiple variants into an additive model and explored the association between the polygenic scores and phenotypes. To test the performance of the polygenic scoring method, we built 100 models at different p-value thresholds by including different sets of variants. Scores distribution at some p-value thresholds deviated from the normal distribution (Shapiro-Wilk $p < 0.05$). Interestingly, we found that the models at these p-value thresholds significantly correlated with the higher values of the variance explained (R^2). We tested each model against the phenotype by means of the linear regression, the model with the highest R^2 (best-fitting) was found at the threshold $p = 0.0742$ and included 49,105 variants. The scores built within this model were significantly associated with the phenotype ($p = 0.00012$).

The present study has several limitations. Firstly, as mentioned above, the study cohort (171 individuals in total, 165 individuals after the quality control) has a limited power to establish significant single variant association and we were observing only a set of suggestively associated variants. Secondly, due to the lack of an external GWAS summary statistics for the same phenotype, we divided our cohort into discovery and target group. Though we performed 1000 random sampling iterations and averaged the resulting scores for each threshold, the risk of overfitting may still be present. The growth of the sample size of the present cohort as well as the appearance of the similarly designed studies with the summary statistics available will help to overcome the described limitations.

5   Conclusion

The present study performed a single variant analysis (genome-wide association study) and a multiple variant analysis (polygenic score modeling) of the type I muscle fibers proportion. Firstly, we established several suggestive genetic variants (p-value < 0.00001) connected to the phenotype that can be potentially replicated with a larger samples size. Secondly, we found an association between the phenotypes and scores at different p-value thresholds. The best-fitting regression model ($p = 0.00012$) explained 8.7% of the variability.

Acknowledgements. This work was supported by the Russian Science Foundation, Grant No. 17-15-01436: "Comprehensive analysis of the contribution of genetic, epigenetic and environmental factors in the individual variability of the composition of human muscle fibers".

References

Ahmetov, I.I., Vinogradova, O.L., Williams, A.G.: Gene polymorphisms and fiber-type composition of human skeletal muscle. Int. J. Sport Nutr. Exerc. Metab. **22**(4), 292–303 (2012)

Balding, D.J.: A tutorial on statistical methods for population association studies. Nature Rev. Genet. Genet. **7**(10), 781–791 (2006). https://doi.org/10.1038/nrg1916

Borisov, O., Kulemin, N., Ahmetov, I., Generozov, E.: A novel multilocus genetic model can predict muscle fibers composition. In: Lames, M., Saupe, D., Wiemeyer, J. (eds.) Proceedings of the 11th International Symposium on Computer Science in Sport, IACSS 2017, vol. 663, pp. 164–168. Springer, Cham (2018). https://doi.org/10.1007/978-3-319-67846-7_16

Chang, C.C., Chow, C.C., Tellier, L.C., Vattikuti, S., Purcell, S.M., Lee, J.J.: Second-generation PLINK: rising to the challenge of larger and richer datasets. Gigascience **4**, 7 (2015). https://doi.org/10.1186/s13742-015-0047-8

Curtis, D.: Polygenic risk score for schizophrenia is more strongly associated with ancestry than with schizophrenia. Psychiatr. Genet. **28**(5), 85–89 (2018). https://doi.org/10.1097/YPG.0000000000000206

Turner, S.D.: qqman: an R package for visualizing GWAS results using Q-Q and manhattan plots. JOSS **3**(25), 731 (2018). https://doi.org/10.21105/joss.00731

Dudbridge, F.: Power and predictive accuracy of polygenic risk scores. PLoS Genet. **9**(3), e1003348 (2013). https://doi.org/10.1371/journal.pgen.1003348

Euesden, J., Lewis, C.M., O'Reilly, P.F.: PRSice: polygenic risk score software. Bioinformatics **31**(9), 1466–1468 (2015). https://doi.org/10.1093/bioinformatics/btu848

Yang, J., Lee, S.H., Goddard, M.E., Visscher, P.M.: GCTA: a tool for genome-wide complex trait analysis. Am. J. Hum. Genet. **88**(1), 76–82 (2011). https://doi.org/10.1016/j.ajhg.2010.11.011

Body Composition in Athletes: History, Methodology and Computational Prospects

Sergey G. Rudnev[1,2(✉)]

[1] Marchuk Institute of Numerical Mathematics, Gubkin Street 8,

119333 Moscow, Russia

sergey.rudnev@gmail.com

[2] Federal Research Institute for Health Organization and Informatics,
Dobrolyubov Street 11, 127254 Moscow, Russia

Abstract. In this work, current methodology and state of body composition studies in athletes are described. Computer science-related issues and prospects of body composition research are outlined, including that of data collection, comparability, utilization, and management.

Keywords: Body composition · Sport · Athletes · Computer science

1 Introduction

Body composition and physique are well-established determinants of health, nutrition and performance in athletes. There are a number of classical (Tanner 1964; Bashkirov et al. 1968; Carter 1982) and modern books (Stewart and Sutton 2012; Lukaski 2017) and numerous research papers on this topic. The aim of this work was to describe current methodology and results of body composition studies in athletes and to outline some issues and prospects related to computer science.

2 Body Composition Models and Methods

The term 'human body composition' is commonly understood as the structure of body mass. Various representations of body mass as the sum of its constituents are called body composition models. Currently, the body composition methodology relies on the 5-level model of body structure which presents human body at the atomic (elemental), molecular, cellular, tissue-system, and whole-body levels of structural organization, respectively (Wang et al. 1992), see Fig. 1. The first body composition model was proposed by the Czech anthropologist and physician Matiegka (1921). Within the framework of his model, the body mass is represented as the sum of the following four compartments of the tissue-system level: subcutaneous adipose tissue and skin, skeletal muscles, skeleton, and the residue. These compartments are estimated using

© Springer Nature Switzerland AG 2020
M. Lames et al. (Eds.): IACSS 2019, AISC 1028, pp. 159–165, 2020.
https://doi.org/10.1007/978-3-030-35048-2_19

anthropometric predictive formulas. The Matiegka model is now relatively rarely used because of low availability of reference (gold standard) methods of the tissue-system level (i.e., CT or MRI) and lack of translational research that would allow a conversion between levels.

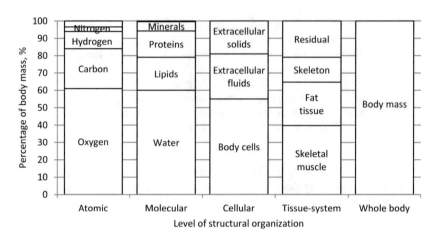

Fig. 1. Structural levels of the body and body composition models (Wang et al. 1992).

The most frequently utilized are body composition models of the molecular level. The conventional two-compartment (2C) model treats body mass as the sum of fat (all lipids) and lean mass (residue) (Siri 1961). Fat and lean mass in the 2C model can be assessed by measuring body density and using assumed densities of fat and lean mass (stable characteristics used as body constants). The reference methods for body density are underwater weighing and air-displacement plethysmography.

One of the conventional three compartment (3C) models can be obtained if consider lean (i.e., fat-free) mass as the sum of dry lean mass and total water content (Siri 1961). In this case, in addition to measuring body density, the isotope dilution method is utilized to access body water, and assumed densities of dry lean mass and body water, are needed. A conventional four compartment (4C) model is obtained in a similar way if consider dry lean mass as the sum of mineral mass and the residue using double-energy X-ray absorptiometry (DXA) for the assessment of body minerals (Selinger 1977). Thus, for the implementation of 3C or 4C models of body composition, some combination of the assessment methods is necessary, such as air-displacement plethysmography, deuterium dilution method and DXA. This model is now considered as a gold standard of body fat estimate and is utilized to check an accuracy of other methods as it takes into account the hydration and mineral status of the body simultaneously.

All in vivo body composition methods, including reference methods, are indirect. The most commonly utilized in athletes are field methods, such as anthropometry and bioelectrical impedance analysis (BIA). Anthropometry and BIA are double-indirect methods since the reference methods, such as air-displacement plethysmography, deuterium dilution, DXA, and 4C model (e.g., a combination of the above three methods) are used for their calibration. The resulting predictive formulas for body composition are population-specific in that they are applicable to individuals of a certain age, sex, ethnicity and physical activity level. Compared to the reference methods, anthropometry and BIA are less accurate but more accessible, less time consuming, relatively inexpensive and still informative which led to their widespread use in population studies (Olds 2009) and sports medicine (Moon 2013). Examples of large BIA databases from various countries can be seen in Table 1. BIA data are commonly utilized to generate centile reference tables for anthropometric and body composition parameters (Cole and Green 1992) which is suitable for data standardization in athletes. The reference methods are used relatively rarely, but their application is necessary in validation studies, clinical studies and research.

Table 1. Large BIA databases: examples.

Country	Data source	BIA instrument	Years of data collection	Sample size	Age interval, years	Reference
China	China Kadoorie Biobank	Tanita TBF 300 GS	2004–2008	512,891	30–79	(Du et al. 2014)
Germany	Precon-centers, Kiel Obesity Prevention Study	BIA 2000-S, Data Input	Up to 2006	230,337	6–102	(Bosy-Westphal et al. 2006)
Russia	Health centers	ABC-01 'Medas'	2010–2012	819,808	5–85	(Rudnev et al. 2014)
UK	UK Biobank	Tanita BC-418MA	2007–2010	186,975	45–69	(Franssen et al. 2014)
USA	NHANES III	Valhalla 1990B	1988–1994	15,912	12–80	(Chumlea et al. 2002)

A more detailed account of body composition models and methods can be found in (Wang et al. 1992; Heymsfield et al. 2005). New promising assessment methods have been recently developed and validated, such as A-mode ultrasound (Wagner et al. 2016) and three-dimensional laser-based photonic scanning (Koepke et al. 2017).

3   Body Composition in Athletes

Information on body composition in athletes is useful for many purposes, such as sports selection, monitoring of training process, physical conditions and readiness, prognosis of athletic performance, control of weight reduction and gain, assessment of functional asymmetries, nutritional status, health status in rehabilitation period, etc.

Athlete-specific anthropometric and BIA body composition formulas are commonly utilized (Moon 2013; Matias et al. 2016). Many studies are focused on the validity of body composition estimates in various sports using different assessment methods and on the data comparability. For example, the study of elite Serbian athletes showed insignificant differences in the percentage of fat mass assessed with the Tanita BF-662W BIA instrument and Jackson-Pollock formulas based on skinfolds (Ostojic 2006). However, the measured impedance values in athletes may differ significantly depending on the type of BIA instrument (Silva et al. 2019). The same applies to skinfold caliper (Marfell-Jones et al. 2013) and DXA measurements (Plank 2005; Nana et al. 2015) due to yet unresolved problem of mutual calibration of the instruments. Therefore, using the same instrument is highly preferable for body composition monitoring at the individual and group levels.

Recent physical activity, body position during measurements, state of hydration, ambient air temperature, skin temperature and other factors are important variables influencing the results of BIA (NIH 1996). In their study of healthy young men, Nickerson et al. (2018) found that already 40 min after a half-hour workout on a treadmill with a moderate intensity (at 60% of the heart rate reserve), the measured impedance values returned to the normal level. Thus, BIA measurements are possible shortly after training of the moderate intensity (but it is still more expedient to use the time before training). It could be of interest to validate the reliability of these findings in elite athletes. Forced normalization of the impedance parameters after intense training was also observed after application of a 10-minute cold shower (Campa 2019).

The availability of DXA is currently increasing (Nana et al. 2015), and the model characteristics of body composition in various sports using DXA have been published (Santos et al. 2014). However, the interpretation of the DXA data in athletes needs caution, as the DXA was inaccurate in the assessment of seasonal changes of body composition as compared to the above mentioned 4C model (Santos et al. 2010).

Closely related to body composition studies is the assessment of somatotype. The Heath-Carter scheme of somatotyping is now one of the most frequently used (Carter and Heath 1990). Kandel (2017) found that the somatotype was a stronger correlate of Ironman race performance in male athletes ($r = 0.54$, $p < 0.01$) than body composition ($r = 0.26$, $p < 0.01$). The mean somatotype in male athletes was 2.4-5.3-2.3 (balanced mesomorph) while the optimal one was somewhat different: 1.7-4.7-3.1 (ectomorphic mesomorph). Our recent studies in apparently healthy children and adults from the general population (Anisimova et al. 2016; Sindeyeva and Rudnev 2017) showed the usefulness of BIA for automatic evaluation of the somatotype and led to the development of appropriate software (Kolesnikov et al. 2016) thus suggesting potential applicability of this approach in athletes.

In Russia, a significant number of cross-sectional anthropometric and bioimpedance body composition studies and virtually no longitudinal studies in athletes have been conducted. Prospective databases of elite athletes are missing, while the reference methods, such as DXA or 4C model, are not yet utilized. Until recently, the Matiegka tissue-system level body composition model was prevalent despite the unknown accuracy of the respective formulas in general population and in athletes. One of the advantages is the availability of the reference population BIA data for data standardization (Rudnev et al. 2014).

4   Summary and Prospects

The study of body composition in athletes is a dynamically evolved area with rapid accumulation of individual body composition data during the athletic season and beyond which can be used to objectively control training process and readiness. Model characteristics of body composition in athletes are updated on a regular basis due to observed secular trends, changing rules and regulations of sports activities, and the emergence of new sports. One of the challenges is the inconsistency of the data from different assessment methods and types of instruments. Preliminary results suggest comparability of BIA data after cross-calibration of BIA instruments at the group level.

Introduction of new high-tech methods, such as three-dimensional laser-based photonic scanning, and the emergence of large databases requires the development of appropriate algorithms and software. Mathematical modeling of physiological mechanisms underlying body mass regulation could facilitate our understanding of optimal training regimens and nutrition in athletes (see, e.g., Hall 2006; Manore 2015). Also of importance is the development of numerical technologies for high-resolution modeling of body composition measurements (Danilov et al. 2018). Other promising issues of athletic health and performance are structural-functional (Silva 2018) and genetic/genomic associations of body composition which will require the development of relevant models and algorithms.

Acknowledgements. This work was supported by the RFBR grant no. 18-59-94015.

References

Anisimova, A.V., Godina, E.Z., Nikolaev, D.V., Rudnev, S.G.: Evaluation of the Heath-Carter somatotype revisited: new bioimpedance equations for children and adolescents. In: Simini, F., Bertemes-Filho, P. (eds.) IFMBE Proceedings, vol. 54, pp. 80–83. Springer, Singapore-Heidelberg (2016)

Bashkirov, P.N., Lutovinova, N.Yu., Utkina, M.I., Chtetsov, V.P.: Body Structure and Sport. Moscow University Press, Moscow (1968). (in Russian)

Bosy-Westphal, A., Danielzik, S., Dörhöfer, R.-P., et al.: Phase angle from bioelectrical impedance analysis: population reference values by age, sex, and body mass index. J. Parenter. Enteral Nutr. **30**(4), 309–316 (2006)

Campa, F., Gatterer, H., Lukaski, H., Toselli, S.: Stabilizing bioimpedance-vector-analysis measures with a 10-minute cold shower after running exercise to enable assessment of body hydration. Int. J. Sports. Physiol. Perform. **14**(7), 1006–1009 (2019)

Carter, J.E.L.: Physical Structure of Olympic Athletes. Karger, Basel (1982)

Carter, J.E.L., Heath, B.H.: Somatotyping: Development and Applications. Cambridge University Press, Cambridge (1990)

Chumlea, W.C., Guo, S.S., Kuczmarski, R.J., et al.: Body composition estimates from NHANES III bioelectrical impedance data. Int. J. Obes. **26**(12), 1596–1609 (2002)

Cole, T.J., Green, P.J.: Smoothing reference centile curves: the LMS method and penalized likelihood. Stat. Med. **11**(10), 1305–1319 (1992)

Danilov, A.A., Rudnev, S.G., Vassilevski, Y.V.: Numerical basics of bioimpedance measurements. In: Simini, F., Bertemes-Filho, P. (eds.) Bioimpedance in Biomedical Applications and Research, pp. 117–135. Springer, New York (2018)

Du, H., Li, L., Whitlock, G., et al.: Patterns and socio-demographic correlates of domain-specific physical activities and their associations with adiposity in the China Kadoorie Biobank study. BMC Public Health **14**, 826 (2014)

Franssen, F.M., Rutten, E.P., Groenen, M.T., et al.: New reference values for body composition by bioelectrical impedance analysis in the general population: results from the UK Biobank. J. Am. Med. Dir. Assoc. **15**(448), e1–e6 (2014)

Hall, K.D.: Computational model of in vivo human energy metabolism during semistarvation and refeeding. Am. J. Physiol. Endocrinol. Metab. **291**(1), E23–E37 (2006)

Heymsfield, S.B., Lohman, T.G., Wang, Z., Going, S.B. (eds.): Human body Composition, 2nd edn. Human Kinetics, Champaign, IL (2005)

Kandel, M.: Body shape vs body composition as predictor on Ironman race performance. Int. J. Sports Phys. Edu. **3**(3), 9–15 (2017)

Koepke, N., Zwahlen, M., Wells, J.C., et al.: Comparison of 3D laser-based photonic scans and manual anthropometric measurements of body size and shape in a validation study of 123 young Swiss men. PeerJ **5**, e2980 (2017)

Kolesnikov, V.A., Rudnev, S.G., Nikolaev, D.V., et al.: On a new protocol of the Heath-Carter somatotype assessment using software for body composition bioimpedance analyzer. Moscow Univ. Anthropol. Bull. **4**, 4–13 (2016). (in Russian)

Lukaski, H.C. (ed.): Body Composition: Health and Performance in Exercise and Sport. CRC Press, Boca Raton (2017)

Manore, M.M.: Weight management for athletes and active individuals: a brief review. Sports Med. **45**(Suppl. 1), S83–S92 (2015)

Marfell-Jones, M.J., Stewart, A.D., De Ridder, J.H.: International standards for anthropometric assessment. International Society for the Advancement of Kinanthropometry, Wellington (2012)

Matias, C.N., Santos, D.A., Júdice, P.B., et al.: Estimation of total body water and extracellular water with bioimpedance in athletes: a need for athlete-specific prediction models. Clin. Nutr. **35**(2), 468–474 (2016)

Matiegka, J.: The testing of physical efficiency. Am. J. Phys. Anthropol. **4**(3), 223–230 (1921)

Moon, J.R.: Body composition in athletes and sports nutrition: an examination of the bioimpedance analysis technique. Eur. J. Clin. Nutr. **67**(Suppl. 1), S54–S59 (2013)

Nana, A., Slater, G.J., Stewart, A.D., Burke, L.M.: Methodology review: using dual-energy X-ray absorptiometry (DXA) for the assessment of body composition in athletes and active people. Int. J. Sport Nutr. Exerc. Metab. **25**(2), 198–215 (2015)

Nickerson, B.S., Esco, M.R., Welborn, B.A., et al.: Time course toward baseline of hand-to-foot BIA measures following an acute bout of aerobic exercise. Int. J. Exerc. Sci. **11**(2), 640–647 (2018)

NIH: Bioelectrical impedance analysis in body composition measurement: National Institutes of Health Technology Assessment Conference Statement. Am. J. Clin. Nutr. **64**(Suppl. 3), 524S–532S (1996)

Olds, T.S.: One million skinfolds: secular trends in the fatness of young people 1951–2004. Eur. J. Clin. Nutr. **63**(8), 934–946 (2009)

Ostojic, S.M.: Estimation of body fat in athletes: skinfolds vs bioelectrical impedance. J. Sports Med. Phys. Fitness **46**(3), 442–446 (2006)

Plank, L.D.: Dual-energy X-ray absorptiometry and body composition. Curr. Opin. Clin. Nutr. Metab. Care **8**(3), 305–309 (2005)

Rudnev, S.G., Soboleva, N.P., Sterlikov, S.A., et al.: Bioelectrical impedance analysis of body composition in the Russian population. Federal Research Institute for Health Organization and Informatics, Moscow (2014). (in Russian)

Santos, D.A., Dawson, J.A., Matias, C.N., et al.: Reference values for body composition and anthropometric measurements in athletes. PLoS ONE **9**(5), e97846 (2014)

Santos, D.A., Silva, A.M., Matias, C.N., et al.: Accuracy of DXA in estimating body composition changes in elite athletes using a four compartment model as the reference method. Nutr. Metab. **7**, 22 (2010)

Selinger, A.: The body as a three component system. Ph.D. thesis. University of Illinois, Urbana-Champaign (1977)

Silva, A.M.: Structural and functional body components in athletic health and performance phenotypes. Eur. J. Clin. Nutr. **73**, 215–224 (2018)

Silva, A.M., Matias, C.N., Nunes, C.L., et al.: Lack of agreement of in vivo raw bioimpedance measurements obtained from two single and multi-frequency bioelectrical impedance devices. Eur. J. Clin. Nutr. **73**(3), 1077–1083 (2019)

Sindeyeva, L.V., Rudnev, S.G.: Age- and sex-related variability of the Heath-Carter somatotype in adults and possibility of its bioimpedance assessment (as exemplified by the Russian population of Eastern Siberia). Morfologia **151**(1), 77–87 (2017). (in Russian)

Siri, W.E.: Body composition from fluid spaces and density: analysis of methods. In: Brozek, J., Henschel, A. (eds.) Techniques of Measuring Body Composition, pp. 223–234. National Academy of Sciences, National Research Council, Washington (1961)

Stewart, A.D., Sutton, L.: Body Composition in Sport, Exercise and Health. Routledge, London (2012)

Tanner, J.M.: The Physique of the Olympic Athlete. Allen and Unwin, London (1964)

Wagner, D.A., Cain, D.L., Clark, N.W.: Validity and reliability of A-mode ultrasound for body composition assessment of NCAA division I athletes. PLoS ONE **11**(4), e0153146 (2016)

Wang, Z.M., Pierson, R.N., Heymsfield, S.B.: The five-level model: a new approach to organizing body-composition research. Am. J. Clin. Nutr. **56**(1), 19–28 (1992)

Estimation of Physical Performance Level of Man in Long Space Flight Based on Regular Training Data

Anton V. Eremeev[1], Pavel A. Borisovsky[1(✉)], Yulia V. Kovalenko[1],
Natalia Yu. Lysova[2], and Elena V. Fomina[2]

[1] Sobolev Institute of Mathematics, SB RAS, 13, Pevtsov Street, Omsk, Russia
eremeev@ofim.oscsbras.ru, borisovski@mail.ru
[2] Institute of Biomedical Problems, Russian Academy of Sciences,
76a, Khoroshevskoye Shosse, Moscow, Russia

Abstract. In this paper, we consider the problem of estimation of physical performance level of cosmonauts in long-term space flight, given the data collected during regular locomotor training exercises. The physical performance level of a cosmonaut is measured in terms of "physiological cost" of work, which is calculated as a function of heart rate, running speed and axial load. An algorithm for estimation of the physical performance level, using the data on the regular training on a treadmill is proposed. The algorithm is based on the principles of linear extrapolation and bisection search. The proposed algorithm is tested on the real data measured in the regular training of Russian cosmonauts on board of the International Space Station and compared to a more simple approach and the standard onboard test of physical performance level. The experimental results suggest that the proposed algorithm may be useful for the estimation of the physical performance level of cosmonauts in long-term space flights.

Keywords: Physical performance · Long space flight · Locomotor training · Extrapolation · Bisection

1 Introduction

The main physiological systems that determine human performance at weightlessness are the cardiovascular, respiratory, and motor systems. All of these systems have significant structural and functional rearrangements during space flights [8–10]. Adaptive rearrangements of these systems in microgravity lead to a decrease of physical performance and requires adequate countermeasures in long term space flights. Physical exercise is the main method of maintaining the level of physical performance, functions of the nervous, neuromuscular, bone systems, motor control systems, and orthostatic tolerance in weightlessness [10].

Currently, prevention of decrease of physical performance level of cosmonauts is mainly attained by the locomotor training on treadmill with an appropriate

ⓒ Springer Nature Switzerland AG 2020
M. Lames et al. (Eds.): IACSS 2019, AISC 1028, pp. 166–175, 2020.
https://doi.org/10.1007/978-3-030-35048-2_20

axial load, supervised by experts on the ground [2]. Walk and run on a treadmill demand maintaining the posture, provide adequate sensory stimulation for the tonic muscles, and ground reaction forces comparable with locomotion on the Earth [2]. Axial loading during locomotion is created by a special training-load suit. The total load from the shoulder belts and the belt located on the hips of the cosmonaut determines the amount of load created by the cosmonaut on the treadmill. The axial load is measured as the total applied kilogram-force, expressed as a percentage of body mass.

The first on-board automated system of training process control was developed, based on an expert system [12]. Unfortunately, this system demonstrated unsatisfactory results in Mars-500 on-ground modelling experiments [3]. We expect that a successful development of an on-board automated system requires problem-tailored data analysis methods to process the measurements form daily training, and one of the key parameters is the performance level.

Currently, the performance level of a cosmonaut and the efficacy of countermeasures are estimated by means of a standard treadmill test designated "MO3", which is performed approximately once a month. The performance level of a cosmonaut is measured in terms of the so-called "physiological cost" of work, which is calculated as a function of heart rate, running speed and axial load [2]. Regression analysis of the physiological cost index on the basis of MO3 tests and optimization of training parameters was done in [1].

It is well known that the heart rate is subject to fluctuations, caused not only by the training load and physical state, but also mood and time of the day [4]. Besides that, the measurements of heart rate during the exercise are subject to noise [5] especially onboard the International Space Station (ISS), where radio interference from other equipment may cause additional errors.

The MO3 test puts a significant strain on a cosmonaut, which makes it impossible to perform it frequently. Therefore it is important to develop a method for estimation of physiological cost using the measurements collected during the regular training without the MO3 procedure.

The aim of the current paper is to enable estimation of the performance level of a cosmonaut for effective management of the physical training on board, using *daily* training data on the running speed, treadmill settings, and the heart rate.

Our study involves identification of time intervals for reliable parameters estimation, censoring the input data and extrapolation of the observed measurements to the corresponding values in conditions of the MO3 test. The analysis based on daily physical training data of Russian cosmonauts on board of the ISS indicates that the estimates of the physiological cost obtained from the regular training tend to agree with those computed in the standard onboard MO3 tests. Finally, some similarities and differences in physical performance evaluation and modelling in sports and in conditions of a space flight are discussed.

2   Regular Training and the Standard Performance Test

The Russian program consists of exercises performed twice a day for a total of 150 min daily. Every day the crew members were recommended to use a treadmill

(BD 2) and a cycle ergometer, alternating with the Advanced Resistive Exercise Device (ARED). BD 2 allows two modes of operation: active, i.e., motor-driven, and *passive*, i.e., leg-driven. The passive mode requires more effort than the active mode at any particular speed and axial load level.

Locomotor exercises consist of running and walking on a treadmill, scheduled in a 3-day microcycle. Every day, a training period starts with a passive locomotion and includes two intervals of walking and running [2]. The days of the standard microcycle are illustrated in Fig. 1. Approximately 30 days prior to landing, crew members were advised to perform locomotor exercise two times a day, with the second microcycle identical to the one done on Day 1 in order to increase orthostatic tolerance and vascular tonicity. Also, the microcycle schedule may be modified on some days due to other activities onboard ISS.

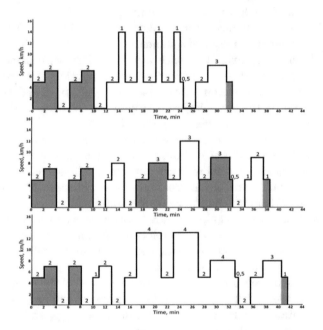

Fig. 1. Three days of the standard microcycle: grey color indicates the passive mode of the treadmill, white color indicates the active mode of the treadmill

The following parameters of locomotor training were evaluated during the exercises on treadmill BD 2: speed in the range of 4 to 20 km/h, weight loading (axial load), the heart rate (using Polar H2), and the treadmill belt mode.

In the long-term missions on ISS, the cosmonaut's performance was monitored on a regular basis. Performance of locomotor exercise was monitored using weekly downloads of the treadmill data. Besides that, several times during the flight the physical endurance of the crew and the efficacy of countermeasures were assessed by means of the standard MO3 test. The MO3 test was carried out when the treadmill functioned in the passive mode and included the following five steps: 3 min of warm-up walk, 2 min of slow running, 2 min of running at a moderate speed, 1 min of running at a maximum speed, and 3 min of cooling-down walk. The sequence and duration of the steps are preprogrammed, but the speed at each stage can be chosen individually. Heart rate (HR), speed, and the axial load levels are the key parameters used for analysis of MO3 results.

In the present paper, the performance capacity at MO3 test is assessed with respect to the physiological cost PhC of work (physiological cost index) calculated as a ratio of heart rate at the end of a running stage HR (bpm) to the running speed of the stage V (km/h) and axial load L (percent of bodyweight):

$$PhC = \frac{HR}{V \cdot L}. \qquad (1)$$

The value PhC is evaluated for the stages of slow running, medium running and fast running. We denote these measurements respectively by PhC_s, PhC_m, and PhC_f. In practice, the most informative indices are PhC_m and PhC_f. Based on the data from the MO3 test, the physical endurance is assessed, and corrections are formulated and uplinked by the flight surgeon, if needed.

3 Methodological Constraints

During a training on Earth, a coach besides the heart rate measurements, is able to evaluate the physical condition of a sportsman and the hardness of an exercise on the basis of visual contact and audio communication with a sportsmen. In the case of workout on treadmill onboard, such sources of information are not accessible to the flight surgeon.

The performance level of a cosmonaut may be calculated as described by the expression (1), where the nominator is the heart rate value. Such choice for the nominator in the physiological cost formula may be seen e.g. in [6]. More often in the recent publications the physiological cost is computed as

$$PhC = \frac{\Delta HR}{V \cdot L}, \qquad (2)$$

where ΔHR is the *heart rate reserve*, i.e. heart rate after load minus heart rate at rest, see e.g. [2]. The heart rate reserve is less sensitive to the individual differences but requires a measurement of the heart rate at rest. In general, the performance indices based on heart rate increase are shown to be a valuable index of performance ability in [11]. However, if the physiological cost of work is predicted on the basis of the daily training, then the heart rate reserve is difficult to estimate since there is no measurement of the heart rate at rest before regular workouts in the current schedule of locomotor training. For this reason, in what follows, we use the physiological cost of work, given by expression (1).

It should be taken into account that during the regular training, a cosmonaut may choose the axial load different from the recommended value due to his/her personal preferences or the current physical state and this setting can be changed in the course of one training session. Besides that, in some stages of the training, the cosmonauts can choose the running speed different from the recommended value. This variability of the axial load and the running speed create a significant difficulty in estimation of physical performance on the basis of regular training.

The heart rate measurements during the MO3 test and during the regular training are subject to fluctuations, caused not only by the training load and physical state, but also mood and time of the day. Besides that, the measurements of heart rate during the exercise are subject to noise. Our preliminary analysis of onboard training data showed that in some cases HR records contain inadequate entries, which may be caused by the radio interference, a lack of contact of Polar with the body or hardware failures. Inadequate high values of HR may also be caused by some physical activity in a time period preceding the considered training period.

4   Estimation of Physiological Cost from Regular Training

In this section, we describe the algorithm for estimation of physiological cost, which, given the data recorded during a one-day regular training period (and maybe several preceding days), computes an estimate of the value PhC for medium speed running stage, as if the MO3 test were performed on this day instead of the regular running exercise. By the definition of PhC, we need the values of axial load, running speed and the heart rate. As it can be seen from Fig. 1, each of the standard three days contains a 10 min. interval in passive mode in the beginning of workout. Such an interval of each training session was the subject of the analysis described in Subsects. 4.4, 4.1. In Subsect. 4.3, we develop a personalized version of the formula for PhC, applicable for a wider range of speed values in comparison to formula (1).

4.1   Search for a Time Interval to Estimate the Physiological Cost

As the MO3 test is performed in passive mode of the treadmill, it is necessary to identify an appropriate time interval I in the first 15 min of a training session.

Finding a Maximum Duration Interval with Speed in Given Range. Given the lower and upper bounds V_{min} and V_{max} for admissible speed values, we can look for the time interval $I_{\max}$, such that only few observations with a speed value outside the range $[V_{min}, V_{max}]$ are allowed, but the total number of such records in the interval should not exceed a threshold of 5%. Another requirement imposed on the time interval $I_{\max}$ is that the entries of HR value outside the allowable range of $[HR_{min}, HR_{max}]$ (boundary values $HR_{min} = 60, HR_{max} = 220$) are allowed, but only up to 10% of the total number of records in $I_{\max}$. The thresholds of 5% and 10% are introduced in order to accommodate some noise, which is present in the measurements of speed and heart rate.

The described algorithm for finding an interval $I_{\max}$ has a drawback that it requires a sufficiently narrow interval $[V_{min}, V_{max}]$, which is hard to define a priori. If the interval $[V_{min}, V_{max}]$ is too narrow, then the identified $I_{\max}$ may be shorter than required for estimation of HR, caused by the running during this interval (e.g. less than 1 min). If the interval $[V_{min}, V_{max}]$ is too wide, then the physical load may change significantly during this interval, which is inconsistent with the MO3 principles and the average speed in this interval does not characterize the training dose properly. As a simple choice for interval I, we can choose $V_{min} = 5$ km/h, $V_{max} = 8$ km/h, attempting to cover the typical range of speed in passive mode onboard training and put $I := I_{\max}$. In the next paragraph, we describe a method for finding V_{min}, V_{max} automatically.

Finding a Time Interval with Small Variation of Speed. For each given workout, we can look for an interval in the passive mode of at least 1.5 min in length with the least variation of speed during the interval. Minimization of speed variation is aimed at finding an interval I with uniform physical load, which would be similar to a 2-min stage of medium run in the MO3 test.

Suppose that a lower bound V_{min} of acceptable speed for interval I is given. We search for the minimal upper bound V_{max}, using the following Bisection Algorithm. This algorithm iteratively reduces V_{max}, while a longest interval with speed in $[V_{min}, V_{max}]$ is at least 1.5 min long. The maximum duration interval $I_{\max}$, where the 95% of speed values are in the range $[V_{min}, V_{max}]$, is found by the procedure described in the previous paragraph. The given value V_{min} remains constant in Bisection Algorithm. The value V_{max} on the input of Bisection Algorithm is set to $V_{min} + 4$ km/h. The iterations of Bisection continue until two consecutive values of V_{max} will differ by at most 0.1 km/h or until a failure to find an interval with speed in range $[V_{min}, V_{max}]$ will occur. The last $I_{\max}$ computed in this algorithm is considered as an output of Bisection Algorithm.

The Bisection Algorithm is called iteratively with $V_{min} = V_{slow}^{med}, V_{slow}^{med} + 0.5, \ldots, V_{med}^{fast}$, where V_{slow}^{med} is the threshold between the slow and medium speed, and V_{med}^{fast} is a threshold between the medium and the fast speed, defined by the available MO3 tests for this cosmonaut (onboard or on Earth). Let V_s, V_m and V_f denote the speed in slow running, medium running and fast running stages of the available MO3 test. Then we define $V_{slow}^{med} := \lfloor V_s + V_m \rfloor / 2$ and $V_{med}^{fast} := \lfloor V_f + V_m \rfloor / 2$. An interval with the least variation of speed, found in the loop over all $V_{min} = V_{slow}^{med}, V_{slow}^{med} + 0.5, \ldots, V_{med}^{fast}$, is returned as the interval I.

Censoring Time Intervals. To exclude inadequate entries in the HR records, we checked that the value HR in the end of interval $I_{\max}$ exceeds the HR value at the beginning of $I_{\max}$ at least by 10 bpm (this is expected as a result of workout).

To avoid undesired high values of HR, caused by high load in preceding time, we checked (i) that the value of HR at the beginning of a training session does not exceed the average initial HR over all training sessions by more than 10 bpm, and (ii) that during a 1-min interval preceding the interval $I_{\max}$, the average treadmill speed does not exceed the average speed of $I_{\max}$ by more than 1 km/h.

4.2   Extrapolation of Heart Rate to the End of 2-min Interval

According to the outline of MO3 test, the heart rate is measured in the end of each 2-min interval of constant load. A preliminary analysis of HR data recorded during MO3 tests indicates that the HR grows nearly linear during each 2-min stage. The duration of the chosen interval I of regular training is usually different from 2 min, therefore, it may be necessary to extrapolate the heart rate to a *supposed* 2-min duration of the interval. Let us assume that the end points of the interval I are t_1 and t_2, i.e. $I = [t_1, t_2]$ and denote $\Delta t := t_2 - t_1$.

If $\Delta t < 2$ min, then HR is extrapolated as follows. Calculate the average heart rate for the first and last 10% of the interval I. These values HR_0 and HR_1 are considered as the heart rate estimates for the moments $t_1 + 0.05\Delta t$ and $t_2 - 0.05\Delta t$. Next, compute the coefficients A, B of a linear function $HR(t) = tA + B$, such that $HR(0.05\Delta t) = HR_0$ and $HR(0.95\Delta t) = HR_1$. Then the heart rate extrapolation to the end of min 2 is computed as $HR(2)$.

In case $\Delta t \geq 2$ min, it is sufficient to compute the average HR starting from the moment $t = 1.9$ min till $t = 2$ min on the interval I.

4.3   Estimation of Physiological Cost at Different Running Speed

Formula (1) was intended to measure PhC_s, PhC_m, and PhC_f, when the cosmonaut is running a particular MO3 stage, and these values can differ significantly in one MO3 test. It is necessary to modify expression (1) for estimation of PhC_m in running with a speed, which may significantly differ from the speed V_m in medium stage of MO3 test. To this end, we substitute V in (1) by a linear expression $a + bV$, where the coefficients a and b are found from the equations

$$\frac{HR_s}{(a + bV_s)L} = \frac{HR_m}{(a + bV_m)L} = PhC_m. \tag{3}$$

Here HR_s, HR_m, and HR_f are the heart rates in slow, medium and fast stages. The three equations given in (3) mean that due to the linear expression $a + bV$ in the denominator, the same value of PhC_m should be found from the data collected in the medium running stage as well as in the slow running stage of the MO3 test, using the new expression

$$PhC = \frac{HR}{(a + bV)L}. \tag{4}$$

4.4   Estimation of Axial Load Recorded During Regular Exercises

In order to censor out the invalid measurements of the axial load, two parameters L_{min} and L_{max} were defined on the basis of the known rules for choosing admissible axial loads during onboard training: $L_{min} = 35, L_{max} = 75$. A preliminary analysis of the registered data showed that, during the exercise, the axial load is sometimes measured with random negative error. In order to reduce such errors in our analysis we consider the maximum value of the observed axial loads in the interval $[L_{min}, L_{max}]$ during the training session. If the training session does not contain any values from the $[L_{min}, L_{max}]$ interval, then the value L is set equal to the axial load in the nearest preceding day when this value was valid, if such a day is found within 10 calendar days (otherwise a workout is discarded).

4.5   Physiological Cost Estimates and the MO3 Results

In order to evaluate the methods proposed in Sect. 4, we carried out a statistical analysis of available data for 14 cosmonauts who participated in long-term space flights. The first MO3 test in each flight was used for computing coefficients a and b by Eq. (3). In the statistical analysis, we computed the correlation coefficient ρ between PhC_m from the second MO3 test in each flight and the PhC estimates based on training sessions. In view of high variability of single-day estimates from training data and frequently missing data (approximately in 10%–30% of the days the valid data were absent), we considered the estimates in each period starting five days before the second MO3 day and ending five days after this day. The PhC estimates from training data in this period were averaged and compared to the PhC_m from the corresponding MO3 test.

Formula (1) applied to the maximum duration interval I_{max} yielded an estimate with $\rho = 0.772$, while the modified formula (4) applied to the interval I found by the Bisection Algorithm yielded an estimate with $\rho = 0.943$. We also performed the Student test for statistical difference in means of the PhC_m at the second MO3 test and the PhC estimates averaged over the closest 5 days as described above. For both of the considered estimates based on the training data, the Student test did not indicate any statistically significant differences, even with significance level $p = 0.1$, i.e. a systematical error is not found.

The physiological cost estimates as well as the values of PhC_m from the onboard MO3 tests for two individuals are illustrated in Fig. 2. It can be seen from the figure that application of the new formula (4) to the measurements from the interval I, found by the Bisection Algorithm, tend to give more accurate estimates of PhC_m than the straightforward application of formula (1) to the measurements in maximum duration interval $I_{\max}$. The coefficients a and b are identified according to (3) on the basis of the first MO3 test in the flight.

5   Discussion

Training on the treadmill onboard ISS has many common features with the training of sportsmen on Earth: In both cases the training dose is carefully measured and recorded, the training schedule is split into micro-cycles, a specific date for achieving maximal performance is given in advance (a competition date for sportsmen and a landing date for cosmonauts), noisy measurements of heart rate during exercises should be taken into account [5], etc. But also some important differences take place. In particular, the amount of training on the treadmill onboard ISS is chosen in such a way that no overtraining should occur. Therefore it is expected that the anaerobic threshold in training onboard the ISS will

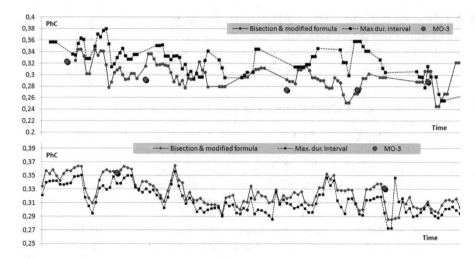

Fig. 2. Results of MO3 test and two estimates of physiological cost: (i) formula (1) applied to the maximum duration interval I_{max} and (ii) the modified formula for physiological cost applied to the interval I found by the Bisection Algorithm. Each node shows an average of estimates for PhC computed in three subsequent days of a flight. The duration of time intervals between the marks on the horizontal axis is 30 days.

not be passed [7], and identification of this threshold is unlikely to be a useful measure of cosmonauts physical performance. Also, it is problematic to measure the blood lactate level onboard, because the procedure of blood collection and its analysis is complicated on the ISS. Therefore the heart rate dynamics during the exercises appears to be the most appropriate source of information about the cosmonauts physical performance level.

6   Conclusions

An algorithm for estimation of the physical performance level of a cosmonaut, using the data on the running speed, axial load and the heart rate in regular training on a treadmill is proposed. The algorithm is based on a modified expression for the physiological cost index and an adaptive search for a time interval, which is similar to one of the stages of the standard MO3 test for physical performance level. Preliminary results of the proposed algorithm suggest that it may be useful for the estimation of the physical performance level of cosmonauts in long-term space flights.

Acknowledgements. The research reported in Sect. 2 is supported by Russian Foundation for Basic Research, project 17-04-01826. The work reported in Sect. 4 is supported by Presidium RAS Program "Basic research for biomedical technologies", project 0314-2018-0001.

References

1. Fomina, E.V., Grushevskaya, U.A., Lysova, N.Yu., Shatov, D.S.: Optimization of training in weightlessness with respect to personal preferences. In: School-Seminar on Optimization Problems and Their Applications (OPTA-SCL 2018) CEUR-WS, vol. 2098, pp. 135–140. RWTH Aachen University, Aachen (2018)
2. Fomina, E.V., Lysova, N.Y., Chernova, M.V., Khustnudinova, D.R., Kozlovskaya, I.B.: Comparative analysis of preventive efficacy of different modes of locomotor training in space flight. Hum. Physiol. **42**(5), 539–545 (2016)
3. Fomina, E.V., Sonkin, V.D., Faletenok, M.V., Zakharov, D.V., Babich, D.R., Surkova, N.Yu., Smoleevsky, A.E., Kozlovskaya, I.B.: Physical training of different direction as the means of profilactics of negative effects of hypomobility in the course of on-ground modelling of interplanetary mission. In: 3rd Symposium of Physiologists of CIS, p. 193. Medicine-Health, Moscow (2011). (in Russian)
4. Hoffmann, K., Wiemeyer, J.: Predicting short-term HR responses to varying training loads using exponential equations. Int. J. Comput. Sci. Sport **16**, 130–148 (2017)
5. Kingsley, M., Lewis, M.J., Marson, R.E.: Comparison of Polar 810s and an ambulatory ECG system for RR interval measurement during progressive exercise. Int. J. Sports Med. **26**, 39–44 (2005)
6. Kozlovskaya, I.B., Yarmanova, E.N., Yegorov, A.D., Stepantsov, V.I., Fomina, E.V., Tomilovaskaya, E.S.: Russian countermeasure systems for adverse effects of microgravity on long-duration ISS flights. Aerosp. Med. Hum. Perform. **86**(12), A24–A31 (2015)
7. Lysova, N., Fomina, E.: Change of aerobic capacity after long duration space flight. In: 42-nd Assembly, 60-th Anniversary, Cospar 2018, Scientific Assembly Program, Pasadena, California, USA, p. 290 (2018)
8. Moore, A.D., Downs, M.E., Lee, S.M., et al.: Peak exercise oxygen uptake during and following longduration spaceflight. J. Appl. Physiol. **117**(3), 231–238 (2014)
9. Norsk, P.: Blood pressure regulation IV: adaptive responses to weightlessness. Eur. J. Appl. Physiol. **114**(3), 481–497 (2014)
10. Shpakov, A.V., Fomina, E.V., Lysova, N.Y., Chernova, M.V., Kozlovskaya, I.B., Voronov, A.V.: Comparative efficiency of different regimens of locomotor training in prolonged space flights as estimated from the data on biomechanical and electromyographic parameters of walking. Hum. Physiol. **39**(2), 162–170 (2013)
11. Sonkin, V.D., Kozlovskaya, I.B., Zaitseva, V.V., Bourchick, M.V., Stepantsov, V.I.: Certain approaches to the development of on-board automated training system. Acta Astronautica **43**(3–6), 291–311 (1998)
12. Son'kin, V.D., Egorov, A.D., Zaitseva, V.V., Son'kin, V.V.: Expert system on managing of physical training of crews in prolonged space flights. Aviokosm. Ekol. Med. **37**(5), 41–46 (2003)

Diagnostics of Functional State of Endothelium in Athletes by the Pulse Wave

Dmitry A. Usanov[1], Anatoly V. Skripal[1(✉)],
Nailya B. Brilenok[1], Sergey Yu. Dobdin[1],
Andrei P. Averianov[2], Artem S. Bakhmetev[2],
and Rahim T. Baatyrov[1]

[1] Saratov State University named after N.G. Chernyshevsky, Astrakhanskaya
Str., 83, 410012 Saratov, Russia
{usanovda, skripalav, dobdinsy}@info.sgu.ru,
brilenoknb@yandex.ru, rahim_baatyrov@mail.ru
[2] Saratov State Medical University named after V.I. Razumovsky,
BolshaiaKazachiastr., 112, 410012 Saratov, Russia
andaveryanov@mail.ru, bakhmetev.artem@yandex.ru

Abstract. The results of diagnosis of the arterial vascular system by the pulse wave recorded by the oscillometric method in a group of athletes engaged in rowing and having high sports categories, as well as the control group have been presented. The reaction of muscle tone to the occlusion of the brachial artery to determine the functional state of the endothelium was studied. To carry out screening diagnostics, we have proposed a method for assessing the functional state of the vascular system by the second derivative of the pulse wave amplitude. The algorithm of the digital signal processing of the pulse wave and the calculation of the index of the functional state of tone of the vascular system of the athletes has been developed. The pulse wave parameters were measured using a software and hardware complex based on the NI ELVIS station. The results of testing athletes for endothelial dysfunction were confirmed by duplex ultrasound scanning of the arterial bed on the device of expert class Philips HD 15 XE. The change in volumetric blood flow after reactive hyperemia was calculated relative to the initial value in two groups of patients. The correspondence between the reduction of the peak value of the volume blood flow obtained by duplex ultrasound scanning of the arterial bed and the reaction to the occlusion of the artery, leading to a decrease in the second derivative of the pulse wave amplitude, measured by the oscillometric method, was shown.

Keywords: Athletes vascular system · Endothelial dysfunction · Pulse wave · Computer biomechanics · Sports medicine

1 Introduction

Current understanding of the state of the cardiovascular system of athletes is based on the fact that the heart and cardiovascular system of athletes differ from the norm [1, 2]. In such athletes, the increase in the volume of blood flow occurs both due to an

© Springer Nature Switzerland AG 2020
M. Lames et al. (Eds.): IACSS 2019, AISC 1028, pp. 176–184, 2020.
https://doi.org/10.1007/978-3-030-35048-2_21

increase in the volume of cardiac output, and due to an increase in the capacity of arterial vessels [3].

Less studied is the question of changes in the functional ability of the vessels of athletes. It is shown [4, 5] that is observed as an increase in vasodilatory capacity of vessels, and the increase in vasoconstrictor tone. At the same time, the changes in the state of arterial vessels in athletes can be both in the direction of increasing the tone and reducing the tone [6].

There are works in which the important role of vascular endothelium in the development of various pathological changes in the functional ability of athletes' vessels is noted [7, 8]. To diagnose the functional state of the endothelium in athletes, various methods can be used based on determining the genetic predisposition of athletes to perform various physical activities [1], measuring the concentration of immunoglobulins of the main classes [9, 10], methods of duplex scanning of arteries [11], measurements of reactive hyperemia index (RHI) and augmentation index (AI) [12].

The development of methods of diagnosis of the arterial vascular system that require a technically complex and expensive system of visualization and measurement of the vascular bed is in conflict with the principles of development of screening diagnostics. In particular, this diagnostics is particularly relevant in assessing the risk of a collapse reaction of the organism to stress and physical activity [12]. Despite the fact that sudden cardiac death in athletes in most cases is associated with sudden cardiac arrest [13], an important role in the development of heart disease can play a change in the functional state of the endothelium of the vascular system of the athlete.

The aim of the work was to substantiate the method of analysis of the arterial vascular system by the pulse wave, recorded by the oscillometric method, and the screening diagnosis of the state of the arterial vascular system on the example of a group of athletes involved in Canoeing and kayaking and having high sports categories.

2 Methods of Measuring the Pulse Wave Shape

To determine the parameters of vascular endothelial function, methods of assessing the elastic properties of arterial vessels during functional tests are used [14]. The most informative functional test is the peripheral vascular occlusion (reactive hyperemia).

From a physiological point of view, the method of occlusion test after removal of pressure in the occlusion cuff causes a sharp increase in the velocity of blood flow in the peripheral channel. With an increase in the rate of blood flow in the brachial artery (BA), the shear stress applied to the surface of endothelial cells increases. This stress leads to the activation of nitric oxide synthesis by endothelial cells, which affects the smooth muscle tone of the artery, changing the shape of the pulse wave.

Currently, there is no unambiguous method for assessing the parameters of the pulse wave shape, which can be used to determine endothelial dysfunction and related pathology of the vascular system. In work [15] for definition of elasticity of vessels the indexes defined as a result of the contour analysis of a pulse wave: reflection index (RI), stiffness index (SI), are used and character of their change at groups of persons of different age is shown. To determine arterial stiffness, a method of volumetric sphygmography [16, 17] is proposed, which allows contour analysis of the pulse wave using a device VaSera VS1000 (Fukuda Denshi, Japan).

To carry out the screening diagnostics, we have proposed a method for assessing the functional state of the vascular system by the second derivative of the pulse wave amplitude from time, by which the risk of cardiovascular insufficiency development under stress was estimated. To register the curvature of the pulse wave in [12, 18], it was proposed to use the parameter P_3 proportional to the second derivative of the pulse wave amplitude.

3   Hardware and Software Complex

The structure of the hardware and software complex includes: desktop workstation NI ELVIS (National Instruments, USA); analog-to-digital Converter (ADC) NI USB DAQmx-device; cuff; rubber pear; monometer; pressure sensor MPX5050GP (Freescale Semiconductor, USA); personal computer or laptop, software kit (LabView 8.5).

The diagnostic procedure included a 10-min rest of the patient, measurement of pressure parameters, fixation of the occlusive cuff on the brachial artery, injection of air in the cuff to the value of diastolic pressure and registration of the pulse shape within 15 s before the occlusion test. At the next stage, the pressure in the cuff was increased by 30–40 mm Hg higher systolic and occlusion was maintained for a period of three minutes. Then the pressure in the cuff was relieved to diastolic, and with the help of a software-hardware complex on the basis of the NI ELVIS station and the pressure sensor MPX5050GP, the pulse wave shape was recorded for 15 s.

4   Data Processing Algorithm

Two groups of 16-year-old patients were selected for the examination: a group of 10 athletes engaged in kayaking and Canoeing, having high sports categories, and a control group, including 10 examined, not suffering from cardiovascular disease. Before the beginning of the diagnostic procedure, each test patient was measured blood pressure on an automatic tonometer and anthropometric indicators (height, body weight). The examination was carried out during the rest of the athletes before the start of training. Measurements of parameters of pulse wave were carried out using software and hardware complex on the basis of the station NI ELVIS (National Instruments, USA). The examination was carried out during the rest of the athletes before the start of training. Written informed consent was obtained from all participants. The study was approved by the Ethical Committee of Saratov State Medical University named after V.I. Razumovsky.

To analyze the pulse wave shape, the amplitude parameter P_3 calculated modulo the second derivative of time d^2A/dt^2 was used [12]:

$$P_3 = \frac{1}{N}\sum_N \left|\frac{d^2A}{dt^2}\right| \tag{1}$$

where A – is the amplitude of the normalized pulse wave (rel. unit), N – the number of points of the pulse wave in which the second derivative was calculated. Parameter P_3 (rel. unit/s^2) was calculated by averaging the values for all cardio intervals of pulse waves. The results of pulse wave signal processing and calculation of P_3 index were displayed by National Instruments LabVIEW 8.5 software (Fig. 1).

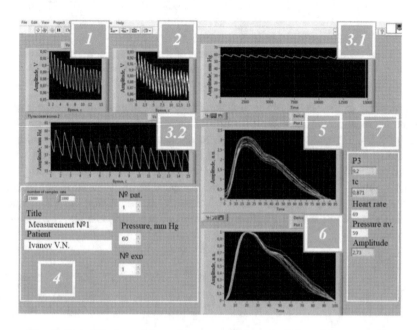

Fig. 1. Data Window of the pulse wave and the calculation of parameter P_3.

Registered signal after passing the DAQmx device and saving in the computer memory was displayed on the graphs of the data output window (Fig. 1) up to 1 and after 2 frequency filtration. After transferring the voltage value to the pressure of the pneumatic sensor, the signal was displayed on the graph 3.1 and 3.2 (the difference in the values along the ordinate axes). In chart 4 (Fig. 1) patient identification data were entered. In window5 all registered cardio intervals are presented. In the window 6 cardio intervals after normalization are shown. In chart 7 the calculated average values of parameter P_3, amplitude, pressure and heart rate were presented.

5   The Results of the Measurement by the Pulse Wave

The results of pulse wave shape measurements for a 16-year-old athlete with the title of candidate master of sports in rowing and Canoeing are shown in Fig. 2: *a*-before occlusion test, *b*-after occlusion test. Calculation of index P_3 of pulse wave before occlusion test was 15.2, and after occlusion test was 12.4.

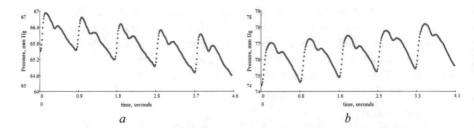

a

b

Fig. 2. Pulse wave 16-year-old athlete with the title of candidate master of sports in rowing and Canoeing: *a*-before the occlusion test (P_3 - 15.2), *b* - after the occlusion test (P_3 -12.4).

According to the results of the analysis, this athlete after a three-minute occlusion test the P_3 index changed in the direction of decrease from the value of 15.2 to the value of 12.4. Thus, there was a reaction to the occlusion of the artery, leading to a decrease in the curvature of the dependence of the pulse wave amplitude on time.

The results of measurements and analysis of the pulse wave shape for a 16-year-old examinee who does not suffer from cardiovascular disease, a member of the control group are shown in Fig. 3: *a*-before occlusion test, *b*-after occlusion test. Calculation of the pulse wave shape index P_3 before occlusion test was 16.9, and after occlusion test was 19.4.

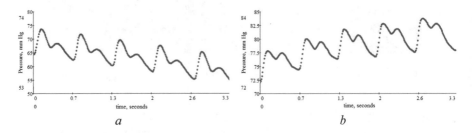

a

b

Fig. 3. Pulse wave of 16-year-old examinee, not suffering from cardiovascular disease: *a* - before occlusion test (P_3 - 16.9), *b* - after occlusion test (P_3 - 19.4).

As follows from the results of the analysis, in the patient from the control group after a three-minute occlusion test, the P_3 index changed in the direction of increase from the value of 16.9 to the value of 19.4. Thus, there was a reaction to the occlusion of the artery, leading to an increase in the curvature of the dependence of the pulse wave amplitude on time (positive reaction of the vascular tone to the occlusion test). The results of measurements of the indexP_3, proportional to the change in the curvature of the dependence of the pulse wave amplitude on time, for the two groups of patients are given in Table 1.

Table 1. P_3 index in two groups of patients before and after the occlusion test

Groups of patients	P_3 index before the occlusion test	Standard deviation σ, %	P_3 index after the occlusion test	Standard deviation σ, %
Athletes	14,1	2,2	11,3	1,7
Control group	15,6	2,4	18,7	1,9

After the occlusion test in a group of athletes, the average value of P_3 decreased by 2.8, while in the control group the average value of P_3 increased by 2.1, which indicates a changed functional state of the vascular tone of athletes with high discharges.

6   The Results of Duplex Ultrasound Scanning

The results of testing athletes for endothelial dysfunction were confirmed by duplex ultrasound scanning of the arterial bed in order to study the dynamics of blood flow rate. For this purpose, Celermajer et al. technique was used, including the study of flow-dependent vasodilation of the brachial artery (endothelium-mediated reaction) [19]. The brachial artery (BA) was visualized in a longitudinal Sect. 5 cm above the elbow bend on an ultrasound device of the expert class Philips HD 15 XE (Netherlands) using a linear sensor (frequency 5–10 MHz).

In the initial state, the internal diameter of BA and the maximum linear velocity of blood flow (Vmax) were measured. Then a three-minute occlusion was performed by compressing the shoulder with a sphygmomanometer cuff placed over the vessel visualization site and creating a pressure exceeding the initial system pressure by 30–40 mm Hg. Immediately after the end of occlusion during the first 30 s Vmax in BA and its diameter were measured. The diameter of the BA was measured at the inner boundary of the artery (intimal layer) at a fixed distance from anatomic landmarks (the surrounding vessel tissue (muscle, fascia)). Then the change of volume blood flow after reactive hyperemia was calculated relative to the initial value. It is considered to be a normal reaction of BA in a test with reactive hyperemia an increase in volumetric blood flow by more than 10% of the initial value [18, 19]. The results of measurements of the peak value of volumetric blood flow of arteries in two groups of patients before and after reactive hyperemia are shown in Table 2.

Table 2. Indicators of endothelium-dependent vasodilation in two groups of patients

Groups of patients	The increase (+) or decrease (−) in the peak values of blood flow, %	Standard deviation σ, %
Athletes	−22%	3,5
Control group	+34%	4,2

After the occlusion test in a group of athletes, the average value of the volume blood flow in the peak decreased by 22%, while in the control group the average value of the volume blood flow in the peak increased by 34%, which also indicates an altered functional state of the vascular tone of athletes with high discharges.

The correspondence of the volume blood flow reduction obtained by the ultrasound method and the response to the artery occlusion, leading to a decrease in the curvature of the dependence of the pulse wave amplitude on time, measured by the oscillometric method, indicate that the method of screening diagnosis of endothelial dysfunction of arterial vessels by the pulse wave has been developed.

7   Conclusion

Currently existing methods of diagnostics of the functional state of arterial vessels are based on the analysis of the amplitude values of the pulse wave or volumetric blood flow. The proposed method is based on the diagnostics of the endothelium of the vascular system by pulse wave shape. The advantage of the method is the use for the diagnosis of information not about the amplitude of the pulse wave before and after the occlusion test, but about the curvature of the pulse wave shape, which is due to the functioning of the muscle tone of the arterial vessels and which is affected by the state of the endothelium.

Comparative analysis of the proposed oscillometric method of screening diagnosis of the arterial vascular system by the pulse wave shape, with the method of duplex ultrasound scanning of the arterial bed was carried out on a group of 10 athletes involved in kayaking and Canoeing, with high sports categories, and the control group, including 10 patients not suffering from cardiovascular disease.

In a group of athletes there was a reaction to the occlusion of the artery, leading to a decrease in the second derivative of the pulse wave amplitude, and in the control group there was a reaction to the occlusion of the artery, leading to its increase. The correspondence between the reduction of the peak value of the volume blood flow obtained by duplex ultrasound scanning of the arterial bed and the reaction to the occlusion of the artery, leading to a decrease in the second derivative of the pulse wave amplitude, measured by the oscillometric method, was shown. At the same time, the proposed method compares favorably with the ultrasound possibility of operative examination of large groups of patients with the help of simple inexpensive equipment that does not require highly qualified personnel for its maintenance.

The conducted studies indicate that a method of screening diagnosis of endothelial dysfunction of arterial vessels to change the shape of the pulse wave before and after occlusion has been developed. Taking into account the possibility of screening diagnostics, it is promising to use it to assess the risk of a collapse reaction of the body to stress and physical activity.

References

1. Green, D.J., Spence, A., Halliwill, J.R., Cable, N.T., Thijssen, D.H.: Exercise and vascular adaptation in humans. Exp. Physiol. **96**, 57–70 (2011)
2. Green, D.J., Spence, A., Rowley, N., Thijssen, D.H., Naylor, L.H.: Vascular adaptation in athletes: is there an 'athlete's artery'? Exp. Physiol. **97**(3), 295–304 (2012)
3. Calbet, J.A., Jensen-Urstad, M., van Hall, G., Holmberg, H.-C., Rosdahl, H., Saltin, B.: Maximal muscular vascular conductance during whole body upright exercise in humans. J. Physiol. **558**, 319–331 (2004)
4. Thijssen, D.H., Maiorana, A.J., O'Driscoll, G., Cable, N.T., Hopman, M.T., Green, D.J.: Impact of inactivity and exercise on the vasculature in humans. Eur. J. Appl. Physiol. **108**, 845–875 (2010)
5. Sugawara, J., Komine, H., Hayashi, K., Yoshizawa, M., Otsuki, T., Shimojo, N., Miyauchi, T., Yokoi, T., Maeda, S., Tanaka, H.: Systemic α-adrenergic and nitric oxide inhibition on basal limb blood flow: effects of endurance training in middle-aged and older adults. Am. J. Physiol. Heart Circ. Physiol. **293**, H1466–H1472 (2007)
6. Kudrya, O.N., Kiriyanova, M.A., Kapilevich, L.V.: Characteristics of peripheral hemodynamics athletes with loads of adaptation to a different direction. Bull. Sib. Med. **11**(3), 48–52 (2012)
7. Al-Alabadi, I.S., Smolensky, A.V.: Genetic aspects of cardiology genetic markers as predictors of sudden cardiac death in sports. Russ. Cardiol. J. **63**(1), 57–61 (2007)
8. Borisov, O.L., Vikulov, A.D.: Vascular endothelial function of athletes. Yarosl. Pedagog. Bull. **1**, 82–85 (2011)
9. Smirnov, I.E., Kucherenko, A.G., Polyakov, S.D., Sorokin, T.E., Bershova, T.V., Bakanov, M.I.: Mediators of endothelial dysfunction during physical strain of the myocardium in young athletes. Russ. J. Pediatr. **18**(5), 21–25 (2015)
10. Green, D.J., Spence, A., Rowley, N., Thijssen, D.H., Naylor, L.H.: Why isn't flow-mediated dilation enhanced in athletes? Med. Sci. Sport. Exerc. **45**, 75–82 (2013)
11. Cioni, G., Berni, A., Gensini, G.F., Abbate, R., Boddi, M.: Impaired femoral vascular compliance and endothelial dysfunction in 30 healthy male soccer players. Competitive sports and local detrimental effects. Sport. Health Multidiscip. Approach **7**(14), 335–340 (2015)
12. Usanov, D.A., Protopopov, A.A., Bugaeva, I.O., Skripal, A.V., Averyanov, A.P., Vagarin, A.Yu., Sagaydachnyi, A.A., Kashchavtsev, E.O.: A device for estimating risk of occurrence of cardiovascular insufficiency during exercise stress. Biomed. Eng. **46**(2), 75–78 (2012)
13. Bokeria, O.L., Ispiryan, A.Yu.: Sudden cardiac death in athletes. Ann. Arrhythmol. **10**(1), 31–39 (2013)
14. Buvaltsev, V.I.: Endothelial dysfunction as a new concept of prevention and treatment of cardiovascular diseases. Int. Med. J. **3**, 202–208 (2001)
15. Kalakutsky, L.I., Fedotov, A.A.: Diagnosis of vascular endothelial dysfunction by contour analysis of pulse wave. Proc. South. Fed. Univ. Tech. Sci. **98**(9), 93–98 (2009)
16. Wang, H., Liu, J., Zhao, H., Fu, X., Shang, G., Zhou, Y., Yu, X., Zhao, X., Wang, G., Shi, H.: Arterial stiffness evaluation by cardio-ankle vascular index in hypertension and diabetes mellitus subjects. J. Am. Soc. Hypertens. **7**(6), 426–431 (2013)
17. Zhou, Z., He, Zh., Yuan, M., Yin, Z., Dang, X., Zhu, J., Zhu, W.: Longer rest intervals do not attenuate the superior effects of accumulated exercise on arterial stiffness. Eur. J. Appl. Physiol. **115**, 2149–2157 (2015)

18. Usanov, D.A., Skripal, A.V., Averyanov, A.P., Dobbin, S.Yu., Kashchavtsev, E.O.: A method of assessing the risk of cardiovascular failure during exercise with the use of laser autodyne interferometry. Comput. Res. Model. **9**(2), 311–322 (2017)
19. Celermajer, D.S., Sorensen, K.E., Gooch, V.M., Spiegelhalter, D.J., Miller, O.I., Sullivan, I. D., Lloyd, J.K., Deanfield, J.E.: Non-invasive detection of endothelial dysfunction in children and adults at risk of atherosclerosis. Lancet **340**, 1111–1115 (1992)

Designing a Mobile App for Treating Individuals with Dementia: Combining UX Research with Sports Science

Bettina Barisch-Fritz[1]([⊠]), Marc Barisch[2], Sandra Trautwein[1],
Andrea Scharpf[1], Jelena Bezold[1], and Alexander Woll[1]

[1] Karlsruhe Institute of Technology, Institute of Sports and Sports Science,
Engler-Bunte-Ring 15, Karlsruhe, Germany
bettina.barisch-fritz@kit.edu
[2] Gustav-Meerwein-Strasse 15, 76228 Karlsruhe, Germany

Abstract. Dementia treatment requires new approaches to delay the progress of the disease. Based on research results to treat dementia a novel approach to combine results from sports science with user experience research (UX) has been taken to develop an application (app) to support hospitalized individuals with dementia by an individualized physical activity program. This paper describes the methodology to develop the app and the current state of the journey.

Keywords: UX research · Dementia · Physical activity · Training in nursing homes

1 Introduction

Dementia is a syndrome of several different types of usually chronic and progressive diseases of the brain affecting the quality of life. The severity of the symptoms and their influence on activities of daily life usually results in permanent care. The number of patients is increasing to approximately 152 million in 2050 [1]. Almost three-quarters of residents in nursing homes have dementia [2]. Therefore, it is valuable to invest into any treatment that delays the disease progression. Physical activity (PA) is promising as some evidence for the slowdown of disease progression is given [3, 4]. Based on the (not yet published) findings of our study [5], the high-aged and differently affected individuals with dementia (IWD) cannot be uniformly treated. Thus, individualized training protocols must be developed based on each cognitive and motor skills.

So far, PA has been instructed either by less qualified employees or by experienced trainers, which is only affordable for selected number of nursing homes. This resulted in huge logistical effort and cost, which cannot be covered by health insurances or individuals. Therefore, an alternative approach for carrying out the training programs by less qualified employees is required.

With the pervasiveness of mobile devices, it was considered that a mobile application (app) is an appropriate way to give access to everybody for adequate testing and training advice. There is variety of factors that decide on the success of the app and in consequence on the positive effects for IWD. Therefore, a novel approach to combine

© Springer Nature Switzerland AG 2020
M. Lames et al. (Eds.): IACSS 2019, AISC 1028, pp. 185–192, 2020.
https://doi.org/10.1007/978-3-030-35048-2_22

sports science with user experience research (UX) is taken to design an app that meets the requirements of different users. The app should be able to test individual cognitive and motor status and consequently provide employees of nursing homes with appropriate individualized training sessions.

This paper is structured as follows Sect. 2 provides background on the state of research for dementia treatment. Section 3 gives an overview on the usage of apps in the area of health and sport science and focuses on apps for IWD. Section 4 covers our approach for the design of a mobile app to simplify dementia treatment within nursing homes. Section 5 concludes this paper and gives an outlook on next steps.

2 Research on Dementia

Dementia has its origin in neuropathological changes that increasingly affect cognitive and motor functions. The current state of research assumes that neuronal cell death and resulting cortical atrophy caused by tangles and plaques are responsible for Alzheimer's disease and similarly circulatory disturbances for vascular dementia [6]. Neuropathological changes of the brain can be identified years before the first clinical signs can be seen [7]. However, not all neuropathological changes lead to the formation of dementia. Thus, there is still a lack within the pathogenesis of dementia. Global research in this field is encouraged and expanded including the treatment of dementia.

Dementia is still incurable, thus a treatment focusing on the delay in disease progression is highly relevant. There is still no effective medicative therapy and the most current backlash of medication research within pharmaceutical industry even questions previous theories on the origin of the disease. This is why non-pharmacological treatment like PA or cognitive stimulation moves into research focus [8].

Previous reviews showed some evidence of PA interventions on cognitive functions [4], motor performance [3], or neuro-psychiatric symptoms like depression [9]. The evidence of PA for IWD is promising, although it is not as clear as the strong evidence within hospitalized elderly persons with other diagnoses [10]. Reasons for the lack of conclusive evidence can be found in small numbers of high-quality studies and diversity of used methods inclusive training parameters [3, 11]. Furthermore, the transfer of knowledge about the generalized positive effects of PA in IWD is unsatisfactory: On the one hand, research findings often provide fragmentary information about training details. On the other hand, there is a lack of adequately trained employees within nursing homes.

3 Mobile Applications in Health and Sports Science

3.1 Applications in Health and Sports

Mobile apps find widespread use and can be found in nearly all areas of life. This phenomenon had its origin with the introduction of Apple's iPhone in 2007. Ten years later, already 2.39 billion smartphone users existed and in 2020 they will further increase to 2.94 billion [12]. Equally, available apps increase (about 254 billion downloaded free apps in 2017) and this industry sector is one of the most growing.

The health and sports sector is one important field for apps. In 2017, 325.000 health apps were recorded [13]. The main focus of these apps is on cardiovascular disease, hypertension, obesity, diabetes, and depression [13]. The specific use cases that different apps address vary widely depending on the interest of the publisher or company. For example, "medication", "diabetes" and "heart, circulation, blood" are main topics from pharma companies, whereas "weight management", or "mental health" are main topics of mhealth app companies, and "hospital efficiency" of hospitals [13].

A systematic literature review presented by Mosa et al. [14] focus on the design, development, evaluation, or use of apps for healthcare professionals, medical or nursing students, or patients. For healthcare professionals with main functions like disease diagnosis, drug reference, medical calculator, literature search, clinical communication, and medical training 57 apps were identified. Eleven apps provide educational material for medical or nursing students and 15 apps directly for patients focusing on management of chronic disease or fall detection [14].

Considering the elderly population with their increasing proportion, health apps have high potential to assist in areas like medication adherence, diabetes management, stroke, or medical care related to falls [15]. 25 health apps were assessed in a systemic review of mobile apps suitable for caring older people [16]. For general drug information, medical references, clinical score, and medical calculator at least two comprehensive mHealth apps exist (Medscape and Skyscape Medical Library). For clinical assessment, diagnosis, drug information, and management of IWD, "Alzheimer's Disease Pocketcard" and "Confusion: Delirium & Dementia" are recommended [16].

3.2 Apps for Dementia

The number of mobile apps that are available in the context of dementia is enormous. Searching the app stores of Apple's iOS and Google's Android operating system for the keyword "dementia" results[1] in 117 and 244 hits, respectively.

In addition to these commercial offerings, there are many scientific publications on apps in the context of Dementia. Various publications address the need to support caregivers with remote monitoring solutions [16] to detect critical situations, like fall detection or tracking the location [17, 18]. There are also approaches to support mental training [19]. Various publications use apps to diagnose dementia and the disease progression. This could either happen by dedicated apps that are used to test disease progression [20] or implicitly by exploiting sensor values provided by smartphones [21]. To the best of our knowledge, there is no app that targets on IWD treatment by PA.

3.3 User Experience Research

UX research became popular in the last decade to develop products and apps that meet user's needs and requirements in the most appropriate way. Instead of developing products based on the knowledge of experts and involving potential customers and stakeholders lately, those are involved throughout the complete product lifecycle.

---

[1] Search conducted on March 22, 2019.

UX research [22] provides a set of tools and methods to investigate users and their experiences systematically to identify requirements for products and apps.

In the field of health apps, utilization of UX is still not common. More often a content analysis approach is adopted [23]. Even if this approach gives information for example about theories or evidence-based practices shaping the app design, it does not reflect the users' perspectives. Considering that after the download of an app only 75% will reopen it [24], acceptance and success of an app is determined by users' interests. Thus, integration of UX into app development can contribute to the effectiveness of an app, as there will be a higher acceptance by end users. However, research is still lacking in this field, as UX is a mainly qualitatively approach. The explorative character of UX might be one obstacle to use it as starting point of app development for scientific purposes. This paper gives an indication how app development can be started with UX methods.

4 UX Design Process

To implement the our app called "inCoPE-App" we have selected the UX design process shown in Fig. 1. It consists of the following phases:

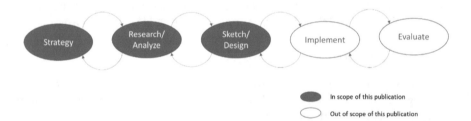

Fig. 1. UX design process

The strategy phase defines long-term goals for the "inCoPE-App" (Sect. 4.1). The phase of research/analysis is used for understanding the prospective users and the actual use cases of the "inCoPE-App. This is essential for the acceptance of the app and thus for successful treatment of IWD. We have conducted a survey, interviews and defined pseudo personas for the definition of user stories (Sect. 4.2).

The sketch/design phase is based on the research/analysis phase. On this base, we started to sketch wireframes. These wireframes will be discussed with potential users and serve as input for the implementation team (Sect. 4.3).

For the implement phase, a professional software development team will realize the "inCoPE-App". The development phase will be divided into two-week sprints. After each sprint, the app can be tested with a set of customers. This phase is out of scope of this paper.

The evaluation phase starts as soon as the app will be used by employees in nursing homes and intends to determine the success of the app. This will happen in two ways: (1) Usage of app: Continuous use of the app to treat IWD is essential for app success.

(2) Positive effects on IWD: If the app will be continuously used, we will be able to evaluate the effects of the training program. This is subject to future work.

4.1 Strategy and Product Vision

Based on previous research we are convinced that PA is beneficious for IWD. In particular, if training sessions can be highly individualized to symptoms and individual needs of each IWD, we expect to achieve a delay in disease progression. The definition of the product vision (Fig. 2) gave a good starting point to align the development of the "inCoPE-App" with the above raised research question.

For employees in nursing homes,
Who treat individuals with dementia
The "inCope-App" **is a** a smartphone-based instruction app for executing training sessions
That proposes individualized exercises for each patient
Unlike traditional training forms that cannot adapt to the individual needs
Our product targets to delay progress of dementia disease and improve quality of life

Fig. 2. Product vision

4.2 Research and Analyze Phase

We rely on the different tools: Observation, Survey and Pseudo personas.
Observations: During our previous research work, we have been in close contact with different nursing homes and got many insights on daily routines of the operative and administrative staff.

Survey: To get an unbiased feedback from employees of nursing homes we defined a questionnaire and conducted interviews with 15 potential users of the "inCoPE-App". The survey resulted in the findings shown in Table 1.

Table 1. Survey findings (15 respondents)

Finding	Description
1	Existence of training manual
	80% of the respondents don't have a training manual to conduct exercises
	93% of the respondents consider a training manual as helpful
2	Structure of training manual
	For 73% of the respondents a good manual in a simple and understandable form is important
	Only 40% of the users consider exercise videos as helpful
3	Content of training manual
	For 80% specific exercises are important
	87% consider education on training sessions as helpful or very helpful

Pseudo personas [25]: Based on our observations (Table 2) and the conducted survey we defined four different pseudo personas presented in Table 3. Each pseudo persona is aligned to one or several real persons we meet in the past. The pseudo personas enable us to analyze and visualize the actual needs of potential users. For example, Fig. 3 shows a typical fictive employee in a nursing home.

Table 2. Respondents' demographics.

Characteristic	Subcategory	Number	Characteristic	Subcategory	Number
Gender	Female	12	Age (years)	31–40	3
	Male	3		51–60	9
Occupation	Director of the nursing home	1		≥ 61	3
	Nursing home manager	1	Origin	Germany	11
	Nursing Staff	3		Italy	2
	Nursing Staff with geronto-psychiatric qualification	2		Tanzania	1
	Additional nursing staff	5		Vietnam	1
	Occupational therapist	1	Main Language	German (beside others)	13
	Sports scientist	1		Swahili	1
	Trainee	1		Vietnamese	1
Total number of respondents		15			

Table 3. Overview on pseudo personas

Person	Role	Age
Giovanna	Full-time nurse	55
Felix	Trainee, supports full-time nurses	18
Eckhard	Director of nursing home	45
Sandra	Sports scientist	34

4.3 Sketch and Design Phase

The get early feedback from potential users we sketched a couple of wireframes that give a good impression how the app will look like. These wireframes have been created with a tool called Balsamiq Wireframes by Balsamiq Inc.

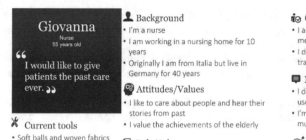

Fig. 3. Example for pseudo person

5 Conclusions and Outlook

The UX research approach gave us many insights on how an app must look like to support employees in nursing homes. When the app will be ready, we will evaluate the impact on IWD. Additionally, we will obtain many additional data for future research.

Essential for design and implementation of apps that handle sensitive patient data is security and privacy protection. Rosenfeld et al. [26] showed that most of the existing apps do not sufficiently address this topic. We will put additional effort on this topic.

Acknowledgements. We thank the Dietmar Hopp Foundation for the support of this project.

References

1. Patterson, C.: World Alzheimer Report 2018. The state of the art of dementia research: New frontiers. Alzheimer's Disease International (ADI), London (2018)
2. Lithgow, S., Jackson, G.A., Browne, D.: Estimating the prevalence of dementia: cognitive screening in Glasgow nursing homes. Int. J. Geriatr. Psychiatry **27**, 785–791 (2012)
3. Blankevoort, C.G., van Heuvelen, M.J.G., Boersma, F., Luning, H., de Jong, J., Scherder, E.J. A.: Review of effects of physical activity on strength, balance, mobility and ADL performance in elderly subjects with dementia. Dement. Geriatr. Cogn. Disord. **30**, 392–402 (2010)
4. Groot, C., Hooghiemstra, A.M., Raijmakers, P.G.H.M., van Berckel, B.N.M., Scheltens, P., Scherder, E.J.A., van der Flier, W.M., Ossenkoppele, R.: The effect of physical activity on cognitive function in patients with dementia: a meta-analysis of randomized control trials. Ageing Res. Rev. **25**, 13–23 (2016)
5. Trautwein, S., Scharpf, A., Barisch-Fritz, B., Niermann, C., Woll, A.: Effectiveness of a 16-week multimodal exercise program on individuals with dementia: study protocol for a multicenter RCT. JMIR Res. Protoc., **6** e35 (2017)
6. The National Institute on Aging NIA: What Happens to the Brain in Alzheimer's Disease? https://www.nia.nih.gov/health/what-happens-brain-alzheimers-disease
7. Villemagne, V.L., Burnham, S., Bourgeat, P., Brown, B., Ellis, K.A., et al.: Amyloid β deposition, neurodegeneration, and cognitive decline in sporadic Alzheimer's disease: a prospective cohort study. Lancet Neurol. **12**, 357–367 (2013)

8. Zucchella, C., Sinforiani, E., Tamburin, S., Federico, A., Mantovani, E., et al.: The multidisciplinary approach to Alzheimer's disease and dementia. a narrative review of non-pharmacological treatment. Front. Neurol. **9**, 1058 (2018)

9. Veronese, N., Solmi, M., Basso, C., Smith, L., Soysal, P.: Role of physical activity in ameliorating neuropsychiatric symptoms in Alzheimer disease: a narrative review. Int. J. Geriatr. Psychiatry (2018)

10. Rydwik, E., Frändin, K., Akner, G.: Effects of physical training on physical performance in institutionalised elderly patients (70+) with multiple diagnoses. Age Ageing **33**, 13–23 (2004)

11. Forbes, D., Forbes, S.C., Blake, C.M., Thiessen, E.J., Forbes, S.: Exercise programs for people with dementia. Cochrane Database Syst. Rev., CD006489 (2015)

12. Statista: Number of smartphone users worldwide. https://www.statista.com/statistics/330695/number-of-smartphone-users-worldwide/

13. Research 2 Guidance: mHealth App Economics 2017/2018. Current Status and Future Trends in Mobile Health. www.research2guidance.com

14. Mosa, A.S.M.: A systematic review of healthcare applications for smartphones. BMC Med. Inform. Decis. Mak. **12**, 67 (2012)

15. Boulos, M.N.K., Wheeler, S., Tavares, C., Jones, R.: How smartphones are changing the face of mobile and participatory healthcare: an overview, with example from eCAALYX. Biomed. Eng. Online **10**, 24 (2011)

16. Berauk, A.V.L., Murugiah, M.K., Soh, C.Y., Wong, T.W., Ming, L.C.: Mobile health applications for caring of older people: review and comparison. Ther. Innov. Regul. Sci. **52**, 374–382 (2018)

17. Helmy, J., Helmy, A.: The Alzimio app for dementia, autism amp; Alzheimer's: using novel activity recognition algorithms and geofencing. In: Proceedings of the IEEE International Conference on Smart Computing (SMARTCOMP), pp. 1–6 (2016)

18. Xenakidis, C.N., Hadjiantonis, A.M., Milis, G.M.: A mobile assistive application for people with cognitive decline. In: Proceedings of the International Conference on Interactive Technologies and Games, pp. 28–35 (2014)

19. Nezerwa, M., Wright, R., Howansky, S., Terranova, J., Carlsson, X., et al.: Alive inside: developing mobile apps for the cognitively impaired. In: Proceedings of the Applications and Technology (LISAT) Conference IEEE Long Island Systems 2014, pp. 1–5 (2014)

20. Wu, J.-Y., Wang, S.-M., Cheng, K.-S., Chien, P.-F.: Computerized cognitive assessment system for dementia screening application, pp. 371–374 (2019)

21. Nieto-Reyes, A., Duque, R., Montaña, J.L., Lage, C.: Classification of Alzheimer's patients through ubiquitous computing. Sensors **17**, 1679 (2017)

22. Pannafino, J.: UX Methods: a quick guide to user experience research methods. CDUXP LLC (2017)

23. Abroms, L.C., Westmaas, L.J., Bontemps-Jones, J., Ramani, R., Mellerson, J.: A content analysis of popular smartphone apps for smoking cessation. Am. J. Prev. Med. **45**, 732–736 (2013)

24. Griffith, E.: More than 75% of App Downloads Open an App Once And Never Come Back. http://fortune.com/2016/05/19/app-economy

25. Gothelf, J., Seiden, J.: Lean UX. Designing Great Products with Agile Teams. O'Reilly, Sebastopol (2016)

26. Rosenfeld, L., Torous, J., Vahia, I.V.: Data security and privacy in apps for dementia: an analysis of existing privacy policies. Am. J. Geriatr. Psychiatry **25**, 873–877 (2017)

Towards a Generic Framework for Serious Games

Josef Wiemeyer[(⊠)] (iD)

Institute for Sport Science, Technische Universität Darmstadt,
Magdalenenstr. 27, 64289 Darmstadt, Germany
wiemeyer@sport.tu-darmstadt.de

Abstract. Serious Games are full-fledged games that aim at accomplishing a double mission: to achieve the serious goal without compromising the experience of playing a game (player experience, PX). To develop high-quality Serious Games, an interdisciplinary approach is required which integrates computer science, technology and design, psychology, and pedagogy as well as insights from the application domain.

So far, only domain-specific frameworks have been proposed for selected application fields. Therefore, the aim of this contribution is to present a generic framework and to demonstrate its usefulness by applying it to the domain of sport.

Keywords: Human action and perception · Game technology · Sensors and interfaces · Player experience · Exergames in sport · Interdisciplinary framework

1 Introduction

Serious Games, i.e., "digital game(s) created with the intention to entertain and to achieve at least one additional goal (e.g., learning or health)" [8, p. 3] have received tremendous interest in recent years. Serious Games are full-fledged games that aim at a dual mission: to achieve the serious goal without compromising the experience of playing a game (player experience, PX).

Essentially, Serious Games can be applied to any "serious" application field such as health, education, tourism, marketing, sport, or science. The development of high-quality Serious Games requires an interdisciplinary approach that integrates computer science, technology and design, psychology, and pedagogy as well as insights from the application domain [8]. So far, attempts to create an integrative framework for Serious Games have focused on domain-specific approaches for selected application fields, such as exercising (exergames), health, and motor learning [12, 16, 22, 33]. These concepts are rather specialized and selective. What is still missing, is a generic framework for Serious Games that can be applied to specific application domains. Therefore, the aim of this contribution is to present such a framework and to demonstrate its usefulness by applying it to the domain of sport. This paper is structured as follows: First, the generic framework is presented, i.e., a modular approach with four modules (generic models, technology and design, specific models of gaming

M. Lames et al. (Eds.): IACSS 2019, AISC 1028, pp. 193–200, 2020.
https://doi.org/10.1007/978-3-030-35048-2_23

and PX, and domain-specific models). Second, this approach is applied to Serious Games in sport.

2 A Modular Approach

Considering the scientific basis of developing, evaluating, and implementing Serious Games, at least four domains can be distinguished (see Fig. 1): human behavior and learning in general, technology and design, game theory, and domain-specific models.

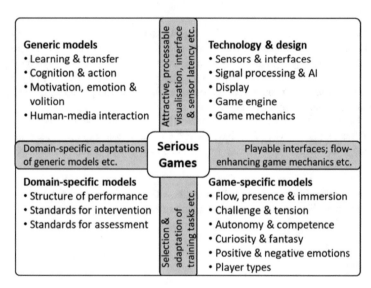

Fig. 1. Modular approach to Serious Games including overlaps of the modules (overlaps: displayed in gray color)

The four modules illustrated in Fig. 1 will be described in the following subsections.

2.1   Module 1: Generic Models of Human Perception and Action

In general, Serious Games aim to change the behavior, skills, knowledge, or attitude of the respective player in a more or less sustainable way. For example, games are designed to help players acquire or improve sensorimotor skills and transfer them into real-life situations. Furthermore, players have to perceive their own actions and the actions of objects or avatars as well as the events in the game, make decisions, control an input device, and so on. Finally, players experience particular emotional and motivational states such as positive and negative emotions, flow, and presence while interacting with the game. Therefore, a consideration and adoption of the respective models contributes to the quality of Serious Games.

Models of human learning cover a wide range of approaches [10]. Basic models of stimulus-response association have been proposed by behaviorism, i.e., classical and instrumental conditioning. These models claim that learning is strongly influenced by (positive or negative) reinforcement. Cognitive approaches focus on the internal processing of information. Computational models, a specific category of cognitive approaches, conceptualize human behavior by means of more or less sophisticated algorithms that are derived from or compatible with insights from psychology and neuroscience. Finally, constructivistic approaches emphasize the importance of authentic learning environments and social interaction.

Models of human cognition and action also cover a wide range of approaches. Models that are often referred to in game research include: self-determination theory (SDT), the theory of planned behavior, and flow theory [8, ch. 2].

Models of emotion, motivation and volition aim at explaining the directedness of human behavior. For example, different types of motivation, such as performance or social motivation, have been proposed to explain why people in similar situations show interindividual differences [32]. Emotions as basic cognitions guiding human approach or avoidance of specific situations comprise at least two dimensions: arousal and valence [26]. Generally accepted emotions are anger, fear, disgust, sadness, and happiness [9]. In Serious Games, fun and enjoyment play a crucial role [20, 31]. Finally, the construct of volition has been introduced to bridge the gap between intention formation and initiation as well as maintenance of human actions [3].

Digital games are a particular type of (interactive) media. Theories of presence and immersion try to explain the process of humans interacting with media [34].

2.2   Module 2: Technology and Design

Technology and design are two closely related fields (see Fig. 1, top right). There are several technology fields that are relevant to Serious Games. When players interact with digital games, they have to operate an interface sensing their movements. Second, the recorded signals have to be classified according to the nature of the player's action or the type of the event. For example, in exergames, the type and parameters of the player's movement have to be identified to trigger the corresponding game response. Third, the game has to be presented by appropriate technologies, e.g., visual displays, speakers, and haptic interfaces. Fourth, the game runs on a stationary or mobile platform with or without connection to the internet.

On the one hand, technology exists that is relevant for, but not specific to, digital games. This technology includes sensors, interfaces, displays, and platforms as well as user interface frameworks and APIs for numerous purposes. In terms of displays, Virtual and Augmented Reality as well as 3D technology offer many options for attractive and effective visualization in Serious Games. When it comes to sensors and interfaces, there is an innumerate field of options available ranging from simple biomechanical or physiological sensors like accelerometers or heart-rate sensors to more or less complex devices like remote controllers, brain-computer interfaces or cameras. With respect to interface design, research has revealed differential effects of interfaces on gameplay and PX [19].

On the other hand, numerous game-specific technologies exist. For example, specific input devices like gamepads or joysticks, and game platforms for mobile and stationary gaming are available. For the development of games, game engines play a crucial role [8, ch. 6]. Modern game engines have a modular architecture that includes a variety of components, for example, gameplay, scripting system, input devices, user interfaces, audio, graphics and rendering, resources, library, and network.

In terms of flexible identification of player behavior and goals as well as control of non-player characters (NPC), data-driven (versus theory-driven) approaches have gained an important role [14, 21]. One important characteristic of data-driven approaches such as machine learning [11, 30] is that classification is rather intuitive than based on explicit a-priori assumptions; however, usually a big amount of valid data is required. A promising approach is to combine theory-driven and data-driven approaches [6].

Game design has a significant impact on the process and results of serious gaming [15]. When designing Serious Games at least two purposes have to be fulfilled [28]: It has to be functional and pragmatic, i.e., allow the players to play the game and reach their goals (effectivity), and hedonic, i.e., elicit and maintain the (emotional) experience of playing, including fun, challenge, curiosity, tension, and emotions (attractivity).

There are numerous generic standards for the design of interactive systems, for example, several ISO standards [2]. The new standards include extended concepts of effectiveness, efficiency, and user satisfaction.

In addition, there are guidelines, heuristics, principles and frameworks for games in general [4] and for the numerous application domains of Serious Games, e.g., exergames [23], or games for cognitive learning in higher education [17].

2.3   Module 3: Specific Models of Gaming and Player Experience

Serious Games are a certain type of games. Therefore, the respective models of gaming and PX are important fundaments of Serious Games (see Fig. 1, bottom right). Gaming or PX is a multifaceted, multidimensional construct [8, ch. 3 & 9]. Two types of models can be distinguished: models of pure gaming and integrative models of Serious Gaming.

Sweetser and Wyeth [29] propose a model of Game Flow that builds on the flow model [25]. The authors claim that eight elements constitute an experience of game flow: concentration on the game, challenges matching the player's skill level, support and development of the player's skills, sense of control over the actions in the game, clear goals, immediate and goal-directed feedback, immersion as deep and effortless involvement in the game, and opportunities for social interaction.

Departing from a user experience model, Nacke [24] proposes a model of PX including seven dimensions: sensory and imaginative immersion, flow, competence, tension, challenge, and positive and negative affects. Based on this model, several questionnaires for the assessment of game (or player) experience have been developed. In addition, several player typologies have been proposed [1]. Finally, integrative models have been developed for specific types of serious games, e.g., for exergames [22, 28].

2.4   Module 4: Domain-Specific Models

The final module addresses the insights in the domain of application. It is of essential importance to include all relevant aspects of the application field into the development of Serious Games. In general, this includes the structure of performance in the respective domain as well as standards for intervention, assessment, and evaluation (see Fig. 1, bottom left).

Taking the example of health, relevant domain-specific knowledge pertains to the three-dimensional concept of health (i.e., physical, psychic, and social well-being), the standards for classification of diseases (e.g., ICD-10), the different categories of health interventions (i.e., primary, secondary, and tertiary prevention, rehabilitation and therapy) as well as specific target groups (e.g., stroke or obese patients). Furthermore, standards for evaluation (e.g. Cochrane or GRADE guidelines) and application (e.g., evidence-based medicine) have to be considered. In addition, numerous national and international laws regulate the application and admittance of medical products.

3   Application of the Framework to the Sport Domain

When developing Serious Games for sport, relevant knowledge regarding the structure of sport performance as well as appropriate learning and training interventions has to be considered in order to influence sport performance in a systematic way. The application of the proposed framework is illustrated by two examples representing the most prominent application fields of exergames in sport: aerobic and balance training.

3.1   Aerobic Training

In this section, the exergame "Exertyfish" is described by applying the proposed framework to aerobic training. Due to the numerous benefits for the human organism, aerobic training is an indispensable part of every training, regardless of performance level. To improve aerobic capacity, there are several training methods available, ranging from constant or variable continuous endurance exercises to intermittent exercises (e.g., high-intensity interval methods). For the application of appropriate training stimuli, the continuous control of training load (stress) and individual training responses (strain) is of great importance. In this regard, heart rate (HR) has often been used as an easy-to-measure parameter representing a reasonable compromise between scientific accuracy and practical applicability [18].

With regard to interface technology, a bicycle ergometer is used for comfortable and controllable indoor training. Furthermore, cadence and HR are measured and work load (braking force) is controlled by employing a bidirectional interface. With respect to design, a natural mapping approach is adopted [27]. The task of the player is to control a fish swimming in a channel, collect rewards and avoid obstacles (see Fig. 2). Pedaling frequency (cadence) affects whether the fish goes up (increasing cadence) or down (decreasing cadence). Control of HR is established by adjusting the braking force of the ergometer. However, because HR shows a delay of one to two minutes in response to the onset or change of training load, appropriate algorithms for predictive HR control have to be developed [13].

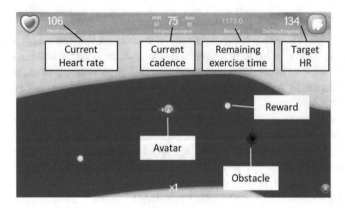

Fig. 2. Screenshot of the exergame "Exertyfish" (legend: HR – heart rate)

Game mechanics and design are chosen to establish a balance between training regimen (effectivity), i.e., keeping HR within certain limits in order to ensure an appropriate training load, and PX (attractivity). To support PX, a simple story, clear goals, immediate and clear feedback, and rewards are deployed [4].

With respect to the adaptation of generic models of human behavior, models of intrinsic motivation, feedback and reinforcement serve as a theoretical basis.

3.2 Balance Training

Balance is an important coordinative ability in sport. In many sports as well as every-day situations, maintaining or reestablishing balance is a prerequisite for successful performance. The most important principle to improve balance is variable training, i.e., the requirements of balance exercise are systematically varied in terms of available information (e.g., eyes open versus eyes closed), time pressure, accuracy pressure, or complexity pressure (e.g., adding dual-task conditions).

A standard in balance assessment is posturography. Participants are located on a force platform to measure postural sway in two dimensions, i.e., medio-lateral and anterior-posterior. The balance board, which operates with four force sensors, is frequently used as choice of game interface in commercial exergames. This interface works quite accurately and closely resembles the methodological standards of the application domain. Furthermore, a natural mapping is established by linking the different directions of weight shifting to the game mechanics, e.g., controlling the direction of a moving avatar by lateral shifts and controlling the speed by leaning back and forth. Another option is to control a maze by weight shifts in the sagittal and frontal plane.

Appropriate PX is elicited by challenging tasks, adaptable task difficulties and reinforcing rewards. Numerous studies have proved that balance exergames are appropriate methods to enhance balance skills, particularly at low initial performance levels [7].

4 Conclusion

The development of Serious Games for specific application domains requires the integration of four modules introduced in this paper. The examples illustrate that considering these modules can support the development of high-quality Serious Games meeting the standards and requirements of the related fields. The framework is also compatible with the three levels of the recently published Serious Games Metadata Format [5].

References

1. Bartle, R.: Hearts, clubs, diamonds, spades: players who suit MUDs. J. MUD Res. **1**(1), 1–27 (1996)
2. Bevan, N., Carter, J., Earthy, J., Geis, T., Harker, S.: New ISO standards for usability, usability reports and usability measures. In: International Conference on Human-Computer Interaction, pp. 268–278. Springer, Cham (2016)
3. Corno, L., Kanfer, R.: Chapter 7: The role of volition in learning and performance. Rev. Res. Educ. **19**(1), 301–341 (1993)
4. Desurvire, H., Wixon, D.: Game principles: choice, change & creativity: making better games. In: CHI 2013 Extended Abstracts on Human Factors in Computing Systems, pp. 1065–1070. ACM, New York (2013)
5. DIN: Serious Games Metadata Format. DINSPEC 91380. DIN, Berlin (2018)
6. Dobrovsky, A., Borghoff, U.M., Hofmann, M.: Applying and augmenting deep reinforcement learning in serious games through interaction. Period. Polytech. Electr. Eng. Comput. Sci. **61**(2), 198–208 (2017)
7. Donath, L., Rössler, R., Faude, O.: Effects of virtual reality training (exergaming) compared to alternative exercise training and passive control on standing balance and functional mobility in healthy community-dwelling seniors: a meta-analytical review. Sport. Med. **46**(9), 1293–1309 (2016)
8. Dörner, R., Göbel, S., Effelsberg, W., Wiemeyer, J. (eds.): Serious Games - Foundations, Concepts and Practice. Springer, Cham (2016)
9. Ekman, P.: What scientists who study emotion agree about. Perspect. Psychol. Sci. **11**(1), 31–34 (2016)
10. Ertmer, P.A., Newby, T.J.: Behaviorism, cognitivism, constructivism: comparing critical features from an instructional design perspective. Perform. Improv. Q. **26**(2), 43–71 (2013)
11. Galway, L., Charles, D., Black, M.: Machine learning in digital games: a survey. Artif. Intell. Rev. **29**(2), 123–161 (2008)
12. Hardy, S., Dutz, T., Wiemeyer, J., Göbel, S., Steinmetz, R.: Framework for personalized and adaptive game-based training programs in health sport. Multimed. Tools Appl. **74**(14), 5289–5311 (2015)
13. Hoffmann, K., Hardy, S., Wiemeyer, J., Göbel, S.: Personalized adaptive control of training load in cardio-exergames - a feasibility study. Games Health J. **4**(6), 470–479 (2015)
14. Hooshyar, D., Yousefi, M., Lim, H.: Data-driven approaches to game player modeling: a systematic literature review. ACM Comput. Surv. (CSUR) **50**(6), 90 (2018)
15. Jabbar, A.I.A., Felicia, P.: Gameplay engagement and learning in game-based learning: a systematic review. Rev. Educ. Res. **85**(4), 740–779 (2015)

16. Kooiman, B., Sheehan, D.D.: Exergaming theories: a literature review. Int. J. Game Based Learn. **5**(4), 1–14 (2015)
17. Lameras, P., Arnab, S., Dunwell, I., Stewart, C., Clarke, S., Petridis, P.: Essential features of serious games design in higher education: Linking learning attributes to game mechanics. Br. J. Educ. Technol. **48**(4), 972–994 (2017)
18. Ludwig, M., Hoffmann, K., Endler, S., Asteroth, A., Wiemeyer, J.: Measurement, prediction, and control of individual heart rate responses to exercise - basics and options for wearable devices. Front. Physiol. **9**, 778 (2018)
19. Martin, A.L., Wiemeyer, J.: The impact of different gaming interfaces on spatial experience and spatial presence – a pilot study. In: Göbel, S., Müller, W., Urban, B., Wiemeyer, J. (eds.) E-Learning and Games for Training, Education, Health and Sports, pp. 177–182. Springer, Berlin (2012)
20. Mellecker, R., Lyons, E.J., Baranowski, T.: Disentangling fun and enjoyment in exergames using an expanded design, play, experience framework: a narrative review. Games Health J. **2**(3), 142–149 (2013)
21. Millington, I., Funge, J.: Artificial Intelligence for Games, 2nd edn. CRC Press, Boca Raton (2016)
22. Mueller, F., Edge, D., Vetere, F., Gibbs, M.R., Agamanolis, S., Bongers, B. Sheridan, J.G.: Designing sports: a framework for exertion games. In: CHI 2011: Proceedings of the SIGCHI Conference on Human Factors in Computing Systems. Vancouver, Canada (2011)
23. Mueller, F., Isbister, K.: Movement-based game guidelines. In: Proceedings of the 32nd Annual ACM Conference on Human Factors in Computing Systems, pp. 2191–2200. ACM, New York (2014)
24. Nacke, L. E.: Affective ludology: Scientific measurement of user experience in interactive entertainment. Doctoral dissertation, Institute of Technology, Blekinge, SWE (2009)
25. Nakamura, J., Csikszentmihalyi, M.: The concept of flow. In: Csikszentmihalyi, M. (ed.) Flow and the Foundations of Positive Psychology, pp. 239–263. Springer, Dordrech (2014)
26. Russell, J.A.: A circumplex model of affect. J. Pers. Soc. Psychol. **39**(6), 1161–1178 (1980)
27. Skalski, P., Tamborini, R., Shelton, A., Buncher, M., Lindmark, P.: Mapping the road to fun: Natural video game controllers, presence, and game enjoyment. New Media Soc. **13**(2), 224–242 (2011)
28. Sinclair, J.: Feedback control for exergames. Doctoral dissertation, Edith Cowan University, Mount Lawley, AUS (2011)
29. Sweetser, P., Wyeth, P.: Game flow: a model for evaluating player enjoyment in games. ACM Comput. Entertain. **3**(3), Article 3A (2005)
30. Szita, I.: Reinforcement learning in games. In: Wiering, M., van Otterlo, M. (eds.) Reinforcement Learning, pp. 539–577. Springer, Berlin (2012)
31. Vorderer, P., Klimmt, C., Ritterfeld, U.: Enjoyment: at the heart of media entertainment. Commun. Theory **14**(4), 388–408 (2004)
32. Weiner, B.: Human Motivation. Erlbaum, Hillsdale (2013)
33. Wiemeyer, J., Hardy, S.: Serious Games and motor learning - concepts, evidence, technology. In: Bredl, K., Bösche, W. (eds.) Serious Games and Virtual Worlds in Education, Professional Development, and Healthcare, pp. 197–220. IGI Global, Heshey (2013)
34. Wirth, W., Hartmann, T., Böcking, S., Vorderer, P., Klimmt, C., Schramm, H., Saari, T., Laarni, J., Ravaja, N., Gouveia, F.R., Biocca, F., Sacau, A., Jäncke, L., Baumgartner, T., Jäncke, P.: A process model of the formation of spatial presence experience. Media Psychol. **9**, 493–525 (2007)

Visual Perception of Robot Movements – How Much Information Is Required?

Gerrit Kollegger[1]([⊠]) [iD], Marco Ewerton[2] [iD], Josef Wiemeyer[1] [iD], and Jan Peters[2] [iD]

[1] Institute for Sport Science, Technische Universität Darmstadt, Magdalenenstr. 27, 64289 Darmstadt, Germany
kollegger@sport.tu-darmstadt.de

[2] Intelligent Autonomous Systems, Computer Science Department, Technische Universität, Hochschulstr. 10, 64289 Darmstadt, Germany

Abstract. Human-robot interactions are steadily increasing in all areas of life. In this context, a common motion learning process of human-robot dyads has not been studied so far.

The observation of movement characteristics plays a crucial role in the assessment and learning of movements in human-human dyads. But what visual information of a robot movement can be perceived and predicted by humans?

The following study examines the perception and prediction of robot putt movements by humans with different visual stimuli. Relevant clues could be identified for the specific movement. Ultimately, with sufficient visual information, humans are able to correctly predict the outcome of a robot putt movement.

Keywords: Human-robot-interaction · Dyad-learning · Motor learning

1 Introduction

In recent years, the number of human-robot interactions has increased in numerous areas, e.g. in rehabilitation, in industry or in sport. While robots and humans are often assigned to separate areas, the overlap of work spaces between robots and humans is constantly growing. An important question is how robots and humans can work together effectively. In an ideal cooperative scenario, the perceptions and actions of humans and robots are perfectly matched. In this article we focus on human perception of robot movements.

Numerous studies have shown that even with few stimuli humans are able to perceive and classify biological movements [7]. Based on these results, Runeson developed the "Kinematics Specify Dynamics" Principle [9, 10]. Ballreich was able to show that the kinematics and kinetics of a jump movement could be correctly classified, but not the joint angles [1]. Cañal-Bruland and Williams [2] report evidence that distal cues, e.g. motion of the raquet, play an important role in predicting the directions

© Springer Nature Switzerland AG 2020
M. Lames et al. (Eds.): IACSS 2019, AISC 1028, pp. 201–209, 2020.
https://doi.org/10.1007/978-3-030-35048-2_24

of tennis strokes. Until now, the transferability of the findings for the evaluation of biological movements to non-biological movements has not been considered.

The following study examines how the prediction of the putt length depends on the visibility of various elements of the robot putt, e.g. ball, parts of the robot or club. Depending on the visible elements, different kinematic cues for estimating the robot putt and the resulting putt distances are available to the human observer: First, the speed of movement of robot, club and ball. Second, the speed has a direct impact on the distance the ball and clubhead travel, and the radial distance between them. Third, the duration of the shown video sequences. Due to the higher ball speeds, the duration of the video sequences decreases with increasing putt distance.

2 Materials and Methods

The following describes the method used in the study which is divided into three sub-studies. The sub-studies differ in the presented video sequences.

2.1 Participants

Thirty healthy students (22 males and 8 females), aged 18–26 years, volunteered to participate in three sub-studies. Inclusion criteria was no previous experience with perceptual studies. Demographic data are presented in Table 1.

Table 1. Individual participants characteristics (Mean ± SD) of the sub-studies (sub) and previous experience in G = Golf, R = returning Games, B = ball games and C = computer games.

	N	Gender	Age [years]	Height [cm]	Bodymass [kg]	Handedness [left | right]	Activitys			
							G	R	B	C
sub1	10	1 | 9	20.4 ± 1.8	179.2 ± 6.3	76.3 ± 9.8	0 | 10	0	4	8	8
sub2	10	0 | 10	24.1 ± 1.5	181.9 ± 6.0	78.9 ± 10.2	1 | 9	0	1	6	5
sub3	10	7 | 3	22.6 ± 2.0	170.9 ± 13.0	64.0 ± 17.9	2 | 8	1	6	5	5
Total	30	8 | 22	22.3 ± 2.3	177.4 ± 9.9	73.0 ± 14.3	3 | 27	1	11	19	18

All participants documented their experience (years of exercising and volume in hours per week) in four different groups of activities: (1) golf, hockey and similar; (2) returning games, i.e. tennis, volleyball; (3) ball games, i.e. soccer, basketball; (4) computer-games. Table 2 shows the information provided by subjects regarding their previous experience.

Table 2. Experience in years (y) and hours per week (h/w) in selective sports and computer games (Mean ± SD) per sub-study (sub). Note: Means and SD were only calculated for participants reporting experience.

	Golf and sim.			Returning games			Ball games			Computer games		
	N	y	h/w	N	y	h/w	N	y	h/w	N	y	h/w
sub1	0	0.0	0.0	4	1.0 ± 1.6	.9 ± 1.2	8	11.5 ± 6.8	3.8 ± 2.6	8	7.5 ± 5.7	4.0 ± 4.4
sub2	0	0.0	0.0	1	.9 ± 2.8	.1 ± .3	6	5.9 ± 6.9	2.5 ± 2.4	5	6.8 ± 7.3	3.7 ± 6.2
sub3	1	3.0	2.0	6	2.0 ± 3.7	1.3 ± 1.1	5	2.3 ± 4.1	1.4 ± 1.6	5	5.2 ± 7.2	.9 ± 1.2
Total	1	3.0	2.0	11	3.5 ± 3.3	2.0 ± .7	19	10.3 ± 6.1	4.0 ± 1.7	18	10.8 ± 5.1	4.7 ± 5.1

2.2 Apparatus and Task

As a technical platform for the studies, a BioRob robot arm is used (Fig. 1). This system has four elastically actuated joints. Each joint is connected via four elastic springs with a separate actuator for each joint. The BioRob system was developed specifically for the physical interaction with humans. Due to its lightweight construction the system generates low kinetic energy. The system is safe to use without collision detection. In order to adapt the system to the anthropometric properties of participants, the BioRob arm was attached to a special lightweight frame. This allows easy adjustment of the height and orientation of the robot arm [3, 5, 6].

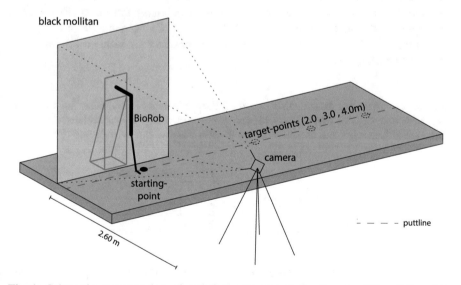

Fig. 1. Schematic representation of technical arrangement for the recording of the video material.

In order to enable a reproducible robot putt and a uniform rolling behavior of the golf balls an artificial putting green was constructed (Fig. 1). The platform is six meters long and two meters wide. The surface consists of a short-pile carpet [3, 8].

The robot putting movements over 3 different putt distances (2.0, 3.0 and 4.0 m) on an artificial putting green were recorded with a Camcorder (Sony FDRAX33) with 50 frames per second. The camera was positioned at a distance of 2.6 m to the ball, perpendicular to the putting direction. As a background, a black mollitan was used, which also covered the mounting frame of the BioRob system (Fig. 1).

The presented video material was produced with Adobe Creative Cloud Premiere Pro CC 2018 (Version 12.0.0). All 12 video scenes had the same basic structure:

1. Preliminary phase: 3 s black screen and two short beeps (duration 0.05 s) after one and two seconds followed by a 1 s freeze frame of the robot in the starting position with a fixation cross centered on the handle and a 1 s beep;
2. Backswing phase: identical motion sequence from starting position to reversal point (duration 0.52 s). Regardless of the putt distance, speed, joint angle, and reversal point were kept constant to avoid spatial cues in this phase;
3. Downswing phase: putt-distance-dependent acceleration profiles from reversal to impact;
4. Follow-through-phase: rolling ball and club motion from impact until the ball passes the right boundary of the image.

For presentation of stimuli the spatial and temporal occlusion technique was deployed [12]. In the processed video material, various areas were removed. Each of the three distances was displayed in six different conditions: full video (FV), hidden robotic arm (HR), hidden robot arm and club shaft (HRC), each in a version with and without ball visible (FVnB, HRnB & HRCnB). Four of the six visual conditions were assigned to each sub-study (Table 3).

Table 3. Assignment of the six conditions to the three sub-studies. Conditions: full video with (FV) and without visible Ball (FVnB), hidden robotic arm with (HR) and without visible Ball (HRnB) & hidden robot arm and club shaft with (HRC) and without visible Ball (HRCnB).

| | Condition | | | | | |
	FV	FVnB	HR	HRnB	HRC	HRCnB
sub-study 1	X	X			X	X
sub-study 2			X	X	X	X
sub-study 3	X	X	X	X		

The video sequences were presented by a self-developed computer program. Video clips were displayed by a projector (EPSON EB-1860, resolution: 1024 × 768px) at the end of the artificial putting green in original size. The projected image of the BioRob system was measured and the projector was set to represent its real size of 1.42 m. Participants watched the video sequences from a distance of 3 m while sitting at a table (Fig. 2).

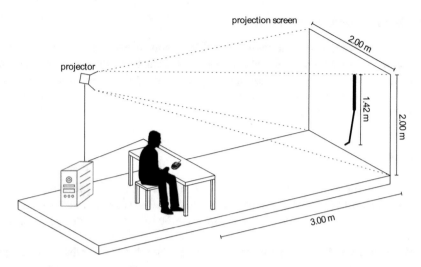

projection screen

projector

2.00 m

1.42 m

2.00 m

3.00 m

Fig. 2. Schematic representation of the experimental setup with the projection screen and the position of the participant.

Each of the 12 video sequences per sub-study were shown four times in randomized order (total of 48 clips). Upon completion of each sequence, a visual continuous analog scale (from 0 to 6 m) was presented to the participants to document their length prediction by clicking on the respective value on the scale with an accuracy of 0.01 m. Following this prediction, participants rated the confidence of their decision on a five-point scale (very unsure, unsure, undecided, sure, very sure).

In addition to the assessment of the putt distance and the confidence, the response/decision time, i.e. time elapsed between the end of the video presentation and the final click on the scale, was also recorded. After assessment, the next video was started by clicking a button. All data was stored by the computer program in one file for each participant.

2.3 Procedure

First, the participants were introduced to the laboratory and the experimental setup by the experimenter. After this introduction, all participants received an informed consent document and a participant questionnaire. After signing the consent and completing the questionnaire, the test software was presented to the subjects and the experimental procedure was described. The participants read the instructions and questions were answered by the experimenter.

After the introductory phase, the participants started the actual experiment autonomously according to the procedure explained in the previous section. After completion of the test program the participants were debriefed.

2.4 Data Processing and Analysis

For each sub-study, a separate two-way ANOVA with repeated measures was calculated with SPSS (V25) with the two factors putt distance (3 distances) and viewing
condition (4 conditions). Wilcoxon tests were applied for follow-up analysis. Bonferroni corrections were applied to multiple comparisons. Level of significance was set
a priori to 0.05.

3 Results

The results of the predicted putt distance in a condensed form, are presented below. In
addition to a descriptive presentation, the results of the ANOVA are also shown. For
reasons of clarity, the results of the distance prediction of the three sub-studies are
summarized.

Means and standard deviations of the predicted putt distance for the three real putt
distances with visible (Fig. 3) and invisible ball (Fig. 4) are illustrated. Short distances
are overestimated, whereas long distances are underestimated.

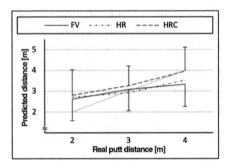 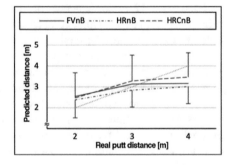

Fig. 3. Real vs. predictet distance in the conditions with ball visible (FV, HR & HRC).

Fig. 4. Real vs. predictet distance in the conditions with ball invisible (FVnB, HRnB & HRCnB).

The predicted distance with the ball visible increases with increasing real distance.
The predicted distance in the three conditions with ball invisible increases initially, but
remains rather constant between 3 and 4 m at a level of 2.84 to 3.45 m.

The two-way ANOVA with repeated measures revealed significant main effects of
distance (all groups), viewing condition (sub-studies 1 & 2) and interaction (sub-study
2), see Table 4.

Table 4. Results of the 3 distances (2, 3 & 4 m) × 4 viewing conditions ANOVA with repeated measures for each of the three sub-studies (VC = viewing condition, D = distance, VCxD = interaction).

Factor	Sub-study 1 (FV, FVnB, HRC & HRCnB)					Sub-study 2 (HR, HRnB, HRC & HRCnB)					Sub-study 3 (FV, FVnB, HR & HRnB)				
	df1	df2	F	p	η_p^2	df1	df2	F	p	η_p^2	df1	df2	F	p	η_p^2
VC	3	27	9,66	<.001	.518	3	27	28.538	<.001	.760	1.699	15.295	.918	.405	.093
D	2	18	24.431	<.001	.731	2	18	43.721	<.001	.829	2	18	15.750	<.001	.636
VCxD	6	54	.235	.963	.025	6	54	4.434	<.001	.330	6	54	1.437	.218	.138

Wilcoxon follow-up analyzes showed consistent differences for the assessment of the putt distance between conditions with and without visible ball, see Fig. 5. Especially for the distances of 3 and 4 m.

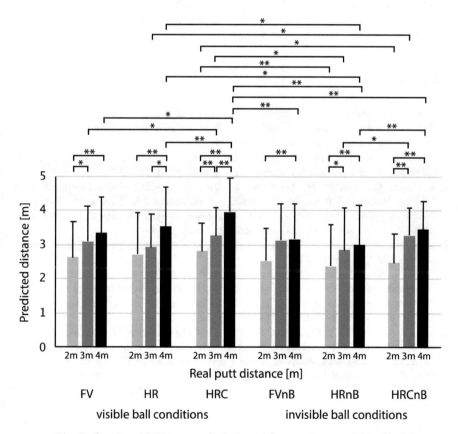

Fig. 5. Results of follow-up analysis for the factors distance and condition.

4 Discussion and Conclusion

The results of the presented study support the current findings regarding the significance of kinematic information, in particular cues derived from the relation of club head and ball movement, e.g. radial distance. The prediction of the putt distance was superior in all conditions with visible ball compared to the conditions without visible ball. These results confirm the special significance of the ball or the relation of club head and ball movement. The robot arm and club shaft do not appear to have a direct impact on the quality of the prediction – possible distractive effect. The reported results are preliminary. Before conclusions can be drawn regarding further studies with adapted optical stimuli, e.g. hidden club head and completely hidden club with visible ball, the respective error scores (AE, CE, VE) must be analyzed [11].

The results confirm previous studies [4]: The putt distance of a robot putt can be predicted by humans based on visual information. In addition, the visibility of the ball has a strong influence on distance prediction. The combination of robot, club and ball adds extra cues to the putt distance, e.g. the variation of the radial distance between the ball and the clubhead at different distances.

References

1. Ballreich, R.: Analyse und Ansteuerung sportmotorischer Techniken aus biomechanischer Sicht. In: Rieder, H., Bos, K., Mechling, H., Reischle, K. (eds.) Motorik und Bewegungsforschung, p. 72–92. Hofmann, Schorndorf (1983)
2. Cañal-Bruland, R., Williams, A.M.: Recognizing and predicting movement effects: identifying critical movement features. Exp. Psychol. 57(4), 320 (2010)
3. Kollegger, G., Ewerton, M., Wiemeyer, J., Peters, J.: BIMROB–bidirectional interaction between human and robot for the learning of movements. In: Lames, M., Saupe, D., Wiemeyer, J. (eds.) Proceedings of the 11th International Symposium on Computer Science in Sport (IACSS 2017), pp. 151–163. Springer, Cham (2018)
4. Kollegger, G., Wiemeyer, J., Ewerton, M., Peters, J.: Visual perception of robot movements. Unpublished manuscript (2019)
5. Lens, T., Kunz, J., Von Stryk, O., Trommer, C., Karguth, A.: Biorob-arm: a quickly deployable and intrinsically safe, light-weight robot arm for service robotics applications. Paper presented at the Robotics (ISR), 2010 41st International Symposium on and 2010 6th German Conference on Robotics (ROBOTIK) (2010)
6. Lens, T., von Stryk, O.: Design and dynamics model of a lightweight series elastic tendon-driven robot arm. Paper presented at the Robotics and Automation (ICRA), 2013 IEEE International Conference on Robotics and Automation (ICRA 2013) (2013)
7. Orgs, G., Bestmann, S., Schuur, F., Haggard, P.: From body form to biological motion: the apparent velocity of human movement biases subjective time. Psychol. Sci. 22(6), 712–717 (2011)
8. Poolton, J.M., Maxwell, J., Masters, R., Raab, M.: Benefits of an external focus of attention: common coding or conscious processing? J. Sport. Sci. 24(1), 89–99 (2006)
9. Runeson, S., Frykholm, G.: Kinematic specification of dynamics as an informational basis for person-and-action perception: expectation, gender recognition, and deceptive intention. J. Exp. Psychol. Gen. 112(4), 585–615.23 (1983)

10. Tremoulet, P.D., Feldman, J.: Perception of animacy from the motion of a single object. Perception **29**(8), 943–951 (2000)
11. Schmidt, R.A., Lee, T.D.: Motor Control and Learning. Human kinetics, Champaign (1988)
12. Wilkins, L.: Vision testing and visual training in sport. University of Birmingham. Ph.D. (2015)

Author Index

© Springer Nature Switzerland AG 2020
M. Lames et al. (Eds.): IACSS 2019, AISC 1028, pp. 211–212, 2020.
https://doi.org/10.1007/978-3-030-35048-2

Printed in the United States
By Bookmasters